THE SURGICAL PATIENT

behavioral concepts for the operating room nurse

THE SURGICAL PATIENT

behavioral concepts for the operating room nurse

BARBARA J. GRUENDEMANN, R.N., B.S., M.S.
Operating Room Nurse Clinician, Centinela Hospital,
Inglewood, California

SHIRLEY B. CASTERTON, R.N., B.S.
Operating Room Supervisor, South Coast Community Hospital,
South Laguna, California

SANDRA C. HESTERLY, R.N., B.A.
Director of Nursing, San Bernardino Community Hospital,
San Bernardino, California

BARBARA B. MINCKLEY, R.N., B.S., M.S., D.N.Sc.
Associate Professor; Assistant Dean, Graduate Programs,
College of Nursing, University of Utah,
Salt Lake City, Utah

MARY G. SHETLER, R.N., B.S.N.
Nurse Epidemiologist, Memorial Hospital Medical Center,
Long Beach, California

SECOND EDITION *with 72 illustrations*

THE C. V. MOSBY COMPANY

Saint Louis   1977

SECOND EDITION

Copyright © 1977 by The C. V. Mosby Company

Previous edition copyrighted 1973

Printed in the United States of America

Distributed in Great Britain by Henry Kimpton, London

The C. V. Mosby Company
11830 Westline Industrial Drive, St. Louis, Missouri 63141

Library of Congress Cataloging in Publication Data

Main entry under title:

The surgical patient.

    Bibliography: p.
    Includes index.
    1. Operating room nursing. 2. Nurse and pa-
tient. I. Gruendemann, Barbara J. [DNLM:
1. Operating room nursing. WY162 S961]
RD99.S95   1977   610.73'677   76-51725
ISBN 0-8016-1981-5

VH/VH/VH 9 8 7 6 5 4 3 2 1

PREFACE
to second edition

Operating room nursing continues to progress. Since the first edition of this book was published, operating room nurses have developed standards of practice that dictate increased responsibility and horizons for nurses in this specialty. The standards also state patient goals—goals that place the patient at the center of all the nurse's activities. This concept is not new; it has always been the hallmark of operating room nursing. The newness is in the formal proclamation, a combination of renewed commitment and human concern.

This second edition incorporates the *Standards of Nursing Practice: Operating Room,* including ideas for implementation of nursing process in the surgical setting. Also included in this edition are new technics and ideas. Each chapter has been carefully analyzed and updated to reflect the current state of operating room nursing.

Behavioral concepts, as the title of the book implies, form the backbone for the second as well as the first edition. It is more difficult to define and quantify behavioral concepts than it is to describe technical procedures. We have, however, continued to develop models for behavioral care of the surgical patient. Sometimes this means "going out on a limb" to crudely describe what we believe is quality nursing care. Our collective experiences with patients have given us many hunches, some of which lack long-term validation by research but nevertheless seem to work in practice. One example is preoperative interviewing by the operating room nurse. Our firm belief is that preoperative contact with the patient has value for both the patient and the nurse. Some research has been done with this practice but not nearly enough.

The second edition contains a certain amount of descriptive material and technical procedures. Any operating room text, behavioral or not, would be incomplete without these. We know that operating room nursing is a combination of doing and thinking and that the nurse must know procedures before she attends to behavioral patient care. Often the care given is a combination of both. So we ask that the reader not isolate the procedures from the other concepts. Both are inherent in high-quality care and cannot be separated from one another.

Operating room nursing does not happen in isolation. More than any other nursing practitioners, those in the operating room constantly work with others and are integral team members. Reading this book is only a first step in improving practice. The proof of the application is at the patient's side—whether circulating, scrubbing, supervising, or teaching. The ultimate result depends on the transfer of knowledge from this book to the operating room. The improvement of practice also comes about by our skill in communicating to others (surgeons, administrators, patients, and families) what it is we do. Operating room nurses have not always done this but have rather assumed that "others know all about us." If our specialty is to progress, we have to assume responsibility for public relations about our work and our philosophy of patient care. Conscious efforts are necessary.

As before, the text is written with both the practicing nurse and student in mind. It has been and can be used as a text in basic nursing programs and continuing education courses for nurses aspiring to be operating room nurses. Seasoned nurses use it as a reference and as a resource for inservice and postgraduate programs.

In this text, nurses are frequently referred to as "she." We did this only for expediency, fully realizing that both men and women are nurses and function equally well. Similarly, many of the patient examples refer to "he"—this was also done for standardization and ease in reading, with full awareness of both female and male patients.

We wish to again acknowledge the cooperation of many people who helped make this book possible: Barbara and Bill Minckley, for the diagrams and drawings; Jill Penkhus, for the anatomic illustrations; Dr. W. E. Mattocks, Ron Zielinski, and Shirley Brooks, for the photographs; those who arranged for and posed for photographs; and the publishers and authors who gave permission to quote from their publications. We are most appreciative.

Barbara J. Gruendemann
Shirley B. Casterton
Sandra C. Hesterly
Barbara B. Minckley
Mary G. Shetler

PREFACE
to first edition

Surgery, to each individual, is a unique experience. Each person perceives and responds to the experience of surgery in a different and unique way. No operative procedure is ever routine, nor can it be labeled "major" or "minor" when a human being is involved.

It is our intent to dispel the idea that the practice of nursing in the operating room is merely a mechanical, technical process. Effective nursing care requires that the patient be seen as an individual and not as a "case." Our endeavor is to stress the importance of the patient as a person or as a friend, and to suggest ways of giving him confidence and a feeling that we, as nurses, are truly interested in him.

The principles of the nurse's role during the surgical procedure will be considered in this book, but they will be discussed in context with the preoperative preparation that has an important effect on the outcome of the surgical experience, and the postoperative phase—a time during which much of the success achieved in both other areas is revealed. We believe that if meaningful nursing care is given in the preoperative and surgical phases of the patient's hospitalization, the postoperative period will reflect this total patient care approach. Experience and evidence have demonstrated that greater understanding and better preparation for the operative experience result in more rapid healing and recovery. Leaving the explanation of the surgical procedure to the physician, the nurse can do much to complement and to explain confusing areas of hospital routine to the patient and his family. It cannot be denied that the family influences the patient's views about surgery and his subsequent recovery. We will suggest methods for better communications between the nurse and family members.

Two assumptions form the basis of this book. First, each surgical patient is unique. Second, certain principles or generalizations can be applied to all surgical patients, asepsis being a case in point. The combination, we feel, forms the basis for *nursing care* of the surgical patient. We are concerned with behavioral concepts and nursing principles that will not only serve the patient in the operating room, but will also be applicable and relevant to patient care in other units of the hospital.

The book is intended as a basic text and reference source for both the nursing student about to approach her surgical nursing experience and the registered nurse, professional or technical, who may see application to her area of practice—the operating room or another nursing unit.

This text is not a "how-to-do-it" procedure manual, nor is it a recipe book of surgical procedures. Procedure manuals are readily available in each hospital to fit that institution's special needs. It is rather a book of selected basic concepts that may be applied to a variety of surgical patients, hospitals, and surgical situations. It was necessary, however, to include a number of "how's" in order to better explain the "why's" which are given primary emphasis.

References throughout the book are to the *operating room (OR) nurse* and the *surgical patient.* The *OR nurse* practices nursing of the *surgical patient,* in or out of the surgical suite. The *OR nurse's* headquarters is the operating room, but her broadening scope of practice includes certain phases of preoperative and postoperative care. We envision the operating room nurse fulfilling a vital role in the continuity of care of the patient undergoing surgery.

Chapter 1 is an introduction to the topic of operating room nursing, to historical anecdotes, and to the importance of nursing theories. The experience of surgery, with implications for both the patient and the OR nurse, is discussed in Chapter 2. Team concepts, nursing responsibilities, and legal and ethical tenets are considered in Chapter 3, Continuity of Care for the Surgical Patient. Chapter 4 includes discussions of nursing histories, nursing diagnoses, and nursing care plans and evaluation. Chapter 5, Development of the Surgical Conscience, contains principles of asepsis, safety, equipment, and medications, as utilized by the nurse when caring for the surgical patient.

Chapters 6 through 9 deal with preoperative, operative, and postoperative nursing care. Explanations and supportive care by the nurse, as well as the role of the family, are included in the chapter entitled Preoperative Nursing Care. Chapter 7, Nursing Care in the Operating Room, contains implications for the nurse, such as receiving the patient, positioning, anesthesia, preparation, tissue differentiation, hemostasis, and instrumentation. Transfer of the patient from the operating room and immediate postanesthesia care, regardless of the type of anesthesia used, are discussed in Chapter 8. The focus in Chapter 9 is on postoperative nursing follow-up, including evaluation of the concept of *care continuity* for the surgical patient. Continuing education, inservice education programs, research, and student education are examined in Chapter 10, Education for Operating Room Nursing.

Our ultimate goal is to reduce the traumatic components of surgery, the "hurts" that need not accompany the patient when he returns home. If the material contained in this text provides one small spark or catalyst in creating a warm, satisfying, professional patient-nurse relationship, our objectives in writing it will have been fulfilled.

We wish to acknowledge the cooperation of many people who helped make this book possible: Barbara and Bill Minckley, for the diagrams and drawings; Jill Penkhus, for the anatomical illustrations; those who arranged for and posed for photographs; and the publishers and authors who gave permission to quote from their publications. We are most appreciative.

B. J. G.
S. B. C.
S. C. H.
B. B. M.
M. G. S.

CONTENTS

THE SURGICAL PATIENT

behavioral concepts for the operating room nurse

CHAPTER 1

OPERATING ROOM NURSING
a theoretical and historical overview

Surgery is a unique human experience. It is unique because it is unlike any other common experience such as eating or sleeping. It is a human experience because it is able to deeply touch, affect, and expose feelings and raw emotions including the fear of pain and death.

Surgery affects the lives of many thousands of people each day. The word *surgery* connotes a plethora of meanings and reactions for each person who has ever undergone such a procedure. It is very difficult to describe accurately a "typical" surgical experience; there undoubtedly is none.

In spite of its individuality, each surgical experience can be planned and managed in a way that assures safety and the most desirable outcome. The scientific knowledge base of operating room nursing is growing and changing. Technologic and humanistic skills are better defined and are being applied to the nursing care of surgical patients. Operating room nurses, using their head, hands, and hearts, have a key role in assisting patients through the events of an operation.

This chapter is an overview of operating room nursing. Trends, historical aspects, and predictions in the field of surgery will be considered, as will the role of the nurse in the patient's surgical course. Selected nursing theories and conceptual models will be analyzed in application to the role of the nurse. Nurse-patient interactions will be emphasized.

We hope that this material will serve as a foundation of thought as the reader proceeds through succeeding chapters. The introductory statements are broad in scope; this is intentional. With this perspective the nurse is allowed more flexibility in individualizing the patient's care.

HISTORICAL REVIEW OF OPERATING ROOM NURSING

Much of the early history of operating room nursing is unrecorded. We can safely assume, however, that at some point in time a surgeon recognized the need for a trustworthy individual to prepare his instruments and materials, assist during operations, and care for equipment afterward. Even though it is difficult to trace the direct progress of this surgical

1

art, we can see that the specialized operating room nurse, or "surgeon's helper," came into being at that time.

Prior to 1900 operations were still being done on any available table. Even so, some of the concepts of surgical nursing were not so radically different from what they are today. For example, surgeon's instruments were boiled before use; food and fluids were withheld; preparations for surgery were made out of the patient's sight; and clean linen cloths were used for drapes. During the operation the "surgical nurse" stood beside the surgeon to hand him instruments and sutures and to sponge up blood as necessary. Postoperatively, the nurse kept constant watch over the patient as he recovered from anesthesia and, in addition, cleaned instruments and burned refuse.

At the turn of the century there came a gradual change in the physical facilities in hospitals. Special areas were set apart for exclusive use as operating rooms. This appears to have marked the beginning of specialization by the surgical nurse. Before this time the nurse had been caring for the patient both pre- and postoperatively in addition to assisting the surgeon during the procedure. But as the number of operations performed and surgeons increased, it became necessary to relinquish pre- and postoperative care of the patient to other nurses. This trend seemed to provide the basis for the separation of the operating room nurse from the other nurses caring for the patient—a separation that is diminishing but still persists in varying degrees. It was not only physical isolation made necessary by the aseptic environment; the isolation was also social.

The early surgical nurse came to function primarily as the surgeon's assistant even before the turn of the century and developed several responsibilities, a primary one being the complete preparation of sutures and sponges. The time-consuming nature of these tasks made it impossible for this nurse to have any responsibility for even rudimentary continuity of patient care. Asepsis was crudely, but carefully, followed in surgery; handwashing was included as a necessary prerequisite to a successful operation.[1]

The following description of the operating room nurse, which is quite sophisticated, was written in 1889:

> A level head, keen eyes, ever watchful for all that may be required, a mind not easily irritated or confused, combined with the faculty of keeping out of the way and still being of the greatest help.*

From the 1920s to the 1940s hospitals were primarily staffed by students. This was also true of the operating room, because an adequate staff of nurses to care for patients was simply not available. Nursing students often spent from 3 to 4 months working in the operating room. Most of their experience was task oriented and geared toward proficiency in clean-

---

*Francis, M. E.: Asepsis for the nurse, The Trained Nurse 3(1):154, July, 1889.

ing and sterilizing gloves and instruments, doing preoperative preps (shaves), and functioning as the surgeon's scrub assistant.

World War II provided a turning point for hospital organization as well as for operating room nursing. Specialization and departmentalization were beginning to reach a zenith. Among other changes, nursing aides and other auxiliary personnel were being accepted as permanent hospital workers. In the operating room change was rapid. Since the supply of nurses was inadequate, a new type of worker, the operating room technician, was introduced. These technicians were enthusiastically accepted by the armed services in World War II and were trained in intensive on-the-job programs. They were found to be capable assistants to the surgeon and functioned in the role of the "scrub nurse." They are still used extensively in many operating rooms, and programs for their training are being standardized and carefully evaluated.

It may have been at this point that operating room nurses began to scrutinize their roles in surgery. Were they really needed as the surgeon's assistant, to pass instruments and prepare sutures, as many novels and television dramas still characterize them today? Concepts began to change as these nurses began to visualize their roles more as leaders, supervisors, and teachers. They saw themselves predominantly as "circulating" or "sponge" nurses, responsible for the overall care of the patient and his environment. The controversy concerning the exact role of the nurse as either the "scrub" or "circulating" person remains today. Most operating room supervisors assess the type of surgical procedure, the surgeon, and the requirements of the patient, and then assign the staff nurse accordingly. Many complex procedures require registered nurses in both scrub and circulating roles, and a knowledgeable scrub nurse can certainly aid the progress of the procedure. The trend, however, seems to be in the direction of putting the registered nurse in the role of leader and coordinator, best exemplified in the position of the "circulating" nurse. This is especially true in operating rooms where the availability of registered nurses is limited and where operating room technicians are employed.

Believing that the circulator during each surgical procedure must at all times be a registered nurse, the Association of Operating Room Nurses formulated a Statement of Policy to this effect. The document speaks to the circulating nurse as the patient's advocate, because of her professional, educational, and practical skills, and because of her physical and social proximity to the patient. The surgeon is in charge of the surgical procedure but relies on the circulator to take charge of the activities of the room and the nursing care required for each surgical patient. The nurse's judgment and professional therapy contribute to a successful operation.[2,3]

Rationale for the mandate is based on the following:

> Patients undergoing surgery experience physical and psychosocial trauma. Not only are most patients unconscious during this time, but they are also completely powerless and unable to make decisions concerning their welfare.

The patient is entering what is probably the most alien environment he has ever known and is removed from the personal contact of family and friends, as well as that of other hospital care personnel. His physical and psychological needs have reached ultimate proportions. At this critical time, patients need much more than technical caretakers; they need professional nurses.*

Roles of the circulating nurse include:

1. Responsibility for nursing activities related to the care of the patient within the operating room
2. Creation and maintenance of a safe and comfortable environment in which surgery can take place
3. Direct and indirect care of the patient, which involves:
   a. Use of nursing judgment and decision making
   b. Knowledge of and ability to use the nursing process in assessing, planning, implementing, and evaluating care
   c. Faculty for effective communication and the ability to recognize and intervene in stress situations involving the patient and/or other team members
   d. Implementation of the principles of medical and surgical asepsis
   e. Current knowledge of the legal implications of surgery
   f. Ability to act in an efficient, rational manner in emergencies
   g. Ability to interact skillfully with and supervise others
   h. Supervision and teaching of members of the surgical team
   i. Acting as the patient's advocate in meeting his physical and psychological needs*

The role of the operating room nurse has recently taken on new dimensions with some added responsibilities outside the operating suite itself. These responsibilities have included pre- and postoperative assessments of the surgical patients by a nurse who is stationed primarily in the operating room (see Chapters 6 and 9). This trend has followed the need for greater continuity of care for the patient. Other benefits are preparatory contact and establishment of rapport with the patient and the ability to collect data and plan for the patient's care. A review of the literature relating to the role of the operating room nurse reflects a beginning awareness of this expanded role and the nurse's responsibility to the patient.[4,5] Operating room nursing should, and indeed can, be truly patient-centered and concerned with human needs. Standards and guidelines have been disvised to incorporate these principles.[6]

THE ROLE OF THE OPERATING ROOM NURSE

The operating room nurse is primarily responsible for the safety and welfare of the surgical patient. Whether conscious or unconscious, the patient must be the center of the nurse's attention.

The operating room nurse teaches, coordinates, and functions as a skilled specialist on the health team. Depending on the patient and the procedure, the nurse may (1) be scrubbed, gowned, and gloved; (2) function

---

*Delegates approve statements, resolutions at twenty-second congress, AORN J. **21**(6): 1068, May 1975. (Reprinted with permission.)

as the manager of a particular operating room; or (3) conduct pre- and postoperative interviews on the surgical unit.

In the operating room the nurse observes the patient's condition and protects him from harm. She anticipates needs and supervises auxiliary personnel and nursing students. The operating room nurse teaches all members of the surgical team aseptic technics, positioning, "prepping," and draping the patient for surgery.

Principles of asepsis must always be applied. The nurse becomes an astute observer of biologic responses while the patient cannot express himself. The nurse, as a problem solver, provides the optimal environment for surgery to take place.

New types of supplies, especially disposables and the latest equipment,

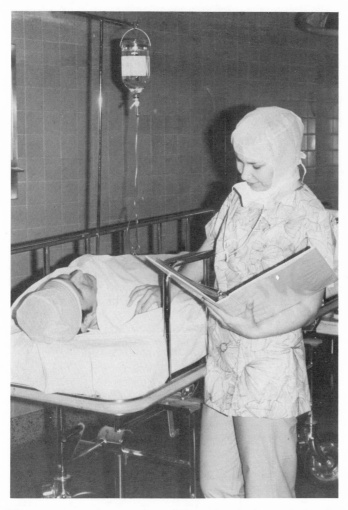

Fig. 1-1. Nurse interacting with patient prior to induction.

are constantly being added to the operating room inventory. In order to utilize these items effectively and efficiently, the registered nurse must be able to demonstrate their use to other members of the health team.

The educational process today deals with the ability to transfer learned concepts and principles to areas of specific action. Many of these concepts are developed to the finest degree in the operating room and once learned can be transferred to any service within the hospital. The most outstanding example of this transferability is the concept of asepsis. In the operating room asepsis must be methodically and conscientiously practiced at all times, whether one is putting away sterile supplies, autoclaving instruments, or opening a room in preparation for a surgical procedure. A set-up cannot be a "little" contaminated. It is either sterile or unsterile. If an unsterile person accidentally touches one corner of a sterile field, the entire area becomes unsterile. When the technic of asepsis is learned in the operating room, it is never forgotten and will be used in other hospital areas such as the delivery room, emergency room, and on the nursing unit when performing aseptic procedures.

The operating room nurse conveys reassurance and identity to the anxious, sedated patient who is awaiting induction of anesthesia (Fig. 1-1). At no other time during his hospitalization is the surgical patient more in need of a feeling of confidence in the health team. His body and life are being entrusted to the team's care. He is totally dependent on others during a surgical procedure.

That the operating room is a critical nursing care area and that the registered nurse is indispensable to the provision of nursing care in the operating room is affirmed by the following resolution:

> The registered nurse has knowledge, experience, and responsibility that prepare her to:
> 1. Independently assess patient needs, therefore implementing nursing intervention
> 2. Make collaborative decisions relative to total intraoperative care
> 3. Make decisions and take action in emergency situations
> 4. Establish and maintain inter- and intradepartmental functioning for continuity of care
> 5. Provide for and contribute to patient safety through control of his internal and external environment, biological testing, and product evaluation
> 6. Assist the patient with the management of anxiety through the application of the principles of biological, physical, and social sciences
> 7. Provide efficient patient care in the operating room through organizational skills, preoperative and postoperative visits, and sound principles of management
> 8. Conduct and participate in research projects directed toward improvement of patient care through the application of scientific principles
> 9. Control hospital costs through budget preparation and implementation
> 10. Participate in architectural design of operating suites effecting efficiency and quality in patient care
> 11. Participate in supervision and instruction of ancillary and allied health personnel in the operating room

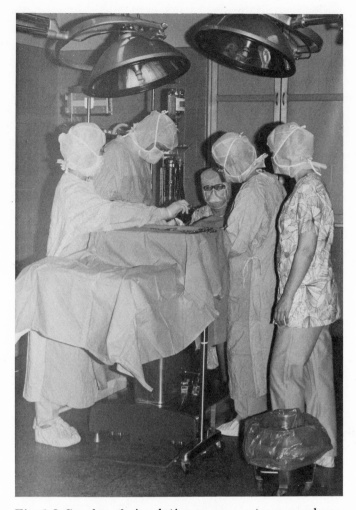

Fig. 1-2. Scrub and circulating nurses as team members.

12. Evaluate and modify the quality of patient care within the operating room.*

As a team leader the registered nurse in the operating room is responsible for organizing, planning, and implementing procedures that aid other surgical team members in performing their functions with a minimum of confusion. In this role the nurse works with members of the team to create a smooth, well-functioning unit (Fig. 1-2). She prepares not only the surgical suite, but also helps prepare the patient for surgery. The operating room nurse plays a vital role in observation and protection of the patient during the procedure.

---

*Necessity for the registered nurse in the operating room, from Delegates approve statements, AORN J. 17(4):188-189, April 1973. (Reprinted with permission.)

A major step of incorporating principles and the concept of nursing process into operating room nursing came with the publication of *Standards of Nursing Practice: Operating Room*. The Standards jointly, developed by the Association of Operating Room Nurses and the American Nurses' Association, provide a model to guide the development of a reliable means of assessing the quality of the nursing process applied to operating room nursing.

According to the *Standards,*

> The *scope* of this practice [operating room nursing] encompasses those nursing activities which assist the individual having surgical intervention. The nursing activities are directed toward providing continuity of care through preoperative assessment and preparation, intraoperative intervention and postoperative evaluation.*

Seven standards enunciate collection of data, nursing diagnosis, nursing goals, planning, nursing actions, implementation, evaluation, and reassessment. The manual is a ready reference for quality nursing care principles.

Unique nursing knowledge in the operating room encompasses caring for the anesthetized patient, providing a safe environment, positioning for proper body alignment, providing psychologic reassurance to the sedated patient, and performing complicated tasks within the sterile environment. In these roles the nurse becomes the agent acting in behalf of the patient throughout the operative experience. This is always the nurse's raison d'etre.

A LOOK INTO THE FUTURE

The technics of surgery are becoming increasingly sophisticated. Operative feats, such as organ transplants, are not only possible, but almost commonplace today. In store for the future will be new and complex equipment, revolutionary concepts, and awe-inspiring results. Surgery will become safer and will be the treatment of choice in a greater number of human conditions and maladies. The number of procedures performed will increase yearly as will the output of those who perform them, the surgeons. This is especially true when one realizes that 60 to 70% of patients who enter general hospitals are coming for surgery.

The treatment and care of surgical patients will remain in the forefront of medicine and nursing for years to come. Trends give no signs for other logical predictions; the incidence of surgery is on the rise. Nursing care of these patients is also becoming more sophisticated and individualized. We now know more about environmental controls and asepsis, but also are becoming more skilled in assessment skills and ways in which psychological

---

*AORN and ANA Division on Medical-Surgical Nursing Practice: Standards of nursing practice: Operating room, Kansas City, Mo., 1975, American Nurses' Association, p. 5. (Reprinted with permission.)

support can be effectively given. The total care concept is sound and popular; it enables nurses to use skills based on scientific knowledge.

When studying growth and trends in surgery, it is important to note not only the increased complexity, but also the *rate* of changes in modes of treatment. Anyone who examines the changes over the past 15 to 20 years and compares them to advances in any other previous time period will find comparisons almost impossible. In looking to the future one can see the difficulty in any attempt at prediction. It can only be said that change will be phenomenal, because change is not only a byword or a cliche; it is stark reality! Because specific procedures and technics will be outmoded a few years from now, nurses and surgeons must be educated in ways of thinking and creating, rather than in set ways of doing.

A future look must also include the emphasis on quality assurance in operating room nursing. Nurses, like other professionals, are becoming increasingly accountable for the care they give. Methods of evaluation of care are becoming sophisticated, patient centered, and outcome oriented. Defining outcomes (or the impact of care on surgical patients) is a difficult task but operating room nurses must be continually asking questions such as: What direct effects does our care have on patients? and Does nursing care make a difference to the patient's eventual outcome? Research is beginning to speak to this issue and to deal with outcomes of care as well as activities of nurses. Audit tools and guidelines (as examples of evaluation) based on the nursing process are being refined and are now used in many hospitals.[7]

THE SURGICAL PATIENT AND THE NURSE

In spite of change, advances, and the varying complexities of surgical treatment, one factor will remain constant—the patient.

Nursing care will vary to accommodate new technical concepts, but the basic nurse-patient relationship will not change, since feelings and attitudes do not change radically simply because of the passage of time. New behavioral approaches will be forthcoming from research; in-depth studies of reactions to surgery may yield more effective ways of nursing the patient with his ever-constant fears and anxieties. These approaches, coupled with new insights into surgical technics, will make nurse-patient interaction increasingly important.

The nurse working with surgical patients has opportunities to affect this human relationship. The nurse can serve as an example and as a source of serenity in the commotion of surgery and can act as catalyst, either to complement the patient process of getting well or to ameliorate the patient process of dying with dignity.

Citizens increasingly demand this type of operating room care. The public has become more vocal in its demand for humanized care. A highly mobile society is asking nurses and other hospital personnel to become more concerned with them as persons and more skilled in talking with them. Close-knit family groups formerly provided the personal contact that seemed to carry a family member through a serious illness. Now relatives often live far away, and the hospital staff may have to serve as a substitute for the family during illness and surgery. Nurses are required not only to be skilled practitioners, but also to be mother surrogates and substitutes for family members who formerly provided personal and physical care to ill members of the family.

The nurse who responds to this human demand while maintaining a high level of skill in technical procedures will be answering a mandate. Technical skills will serve as *means* to the end—patient care—not as ends in themselves. This is the great challenge to operating room nurses and surgical patient care today.

RESEARCH AND NURSING THEORIES

In order to set the stage for a discussion of the role of the operating room nurse, it is necessary to examine the broad generalizations in nursing theory. Theory provides a frame of reference, or ideas, whereby nursing actions may serve a rational purpose. Without the common theoretical framework, nursing care may seem disjointed, purposeless, or generally ineffective. There is also the danger that intuition, or rote ("I've always done it this way"), may become the nurse's steering wheel. A frame of reference or some specified knowledge gives the nurse a basis on which to make decisions about the care that is given.

The material in this book is intended to provide such a frame of reference. This particular section on research and nursing theories is presented early in the text to assist the reader to "digest" the material and to provide frames of reference.

Nursing has taken on new meanings and skills. A wealth of new information can be found in current nursing journals. It becomes necessary, therefore, to select from the readings, to discriminate in our thinking, and to decide on the nursing perspective we wish to adopt. Only when we effectively hold a theory or concept of nursing can we have genuine nursing goals and can we contribute to development in the field of operating room nursing. As Wiedenbach states:

> Answers to questions such as "What is nursing?" and "What is the nurse's unique area of responsibility?" will be found when each nurse identifies for herself the theory that underlies her practice, enunciates it, respects it, and uses it consciously and critically, not just to *guide* her in her practice, but also to serve her as a means to *improve* nursing practice as well.*

Perhaps some analogies will serve to clarify. Members of the United States Congress have guidelines by which their decisions are made. Their political party's platform is one of these guides and is used consciously or

---

*Wiedenbach, E.: Nurses' wisdom in nursing theory, Am. J. Nurs. 70(5):1057, May 1970. (Copyright The American Journal of Nursing Company.)

subconsciously. It is a contributing factor in their thinking. Likewise, the psychiatrist who adheres to a psychoanalytic theory will treat his patients differently from another who holds a behaviorist point of view. Neither of these psychiatrists or congressmen is "right" or "wrong" in his treatment of patients or his political decisions. But, for this discussion, it is important to recognize that each treats or decides *guided by* his thinking, or frame of references. The theory adhered to definitely guides the resultant practices.

The same is true in operating room nursing and in nursing in general. Varying models and modes of giving nursing care are described in almost every nursing journal and nursing text. One perspective of nursing is that of the nurse who serves wholly as the physician's assistant; at the other end of the continuum is the nurse who is an independent practitioner with little direction from members of other disciplines. Nurses concentrate on "why-do-we-do-it?" as well as "how-to-do- it."

An accurate description of nursing theory is elusive and cannot be defined in one sentence. It is a special adaptation of scientific knowledge and, as such, should serve to direct the activities of nursing practice. Theory may help to determine practice, but practice is also essential in developing theoretical concepts in nursing.

Conant dissects nursing theory as she analyzes the practice-theory gap: Pertinent factors must be isolated and described; their relationships must be specified and ordered to prescribe activity that will lead to the desired goal, which also must be specified.* Systematic improvement of practice will come more rapidly when practitioners themselves can integrate research with practice.

Description, explanation, and prediction must be components of a nursing theory. It is perhaps in the stage of prediction and prescription that accurate replicable studies are most needed in nursing today. This is especially true in the area of operating room nursing.

It is difficult to place nursing strictly within a theoretical framework, primarily because it is a *practice* discipline and, as such, involves clinical interaction with patients. Some feel that theory is too abstract to be applicable and practice is too specific to be based on generalizations. Both views are untenable but lead to the most scientifically acceptable tenet: Theory and practice are inseparable and are of equal significance in the formulation of a scientific basis for nursing.

Fig. 1-3 depicts the interrelatedness of theory and generalizations with the specific world of nursing practice. In nursing there is a separation between the two. A true marriage or alliance of these concepts is possible when definitive *nursing* knowledge is delineated to the point of being useful in prediction and control of practice. This goal is the concern of much research today but as yet, has not been fully achieved in nursing.

*Conant, L. H.: Closing the practice-theory gap, Nurs. Outlook 15(11):37, Nov. 1967. 1967. (Copyright The American Journal of Nursing Company.)

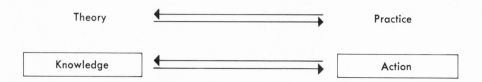

Fig. 1-3. Interrelatedness of theory and practice.

How do research and nursing theory relate to the practice of operating room nursing? For the nurse there is a challenge to observe, clarify, and possibly contribute to a body of knowledge. Questions that an operating room nurse might begin to ask are:

1. If coughing and deep breathing exercises are taught and practiced pre- and postoperatively, does the rate of pulmonary complications decrease?
2. What criteria should be used to administer pain medications postoperatively?
3. What type of explanations should be given to patients preoperatively? Are there patients who would be most comfortable not knowing anything about the operating room, recovery room, or expected course of events?
4. Is the recovery rate affected if one nurse cares for a patient preoperatively, in surgery, and postoperatively?
5. Are measurable postoperative parameters (such as number of medications, length of hospitalization, ability to verbalize, measures of satisfaction versus dissatisfaction) affected by a particular nursing action?
6. Should families automatically be included in preoperative teaching?
7. What are measurable standards of surgical patient health and recovery?

Each practicing nurse and student is able to collect data of varying complexity, compile it, and possibly note some trends or factors that seem to affect patient care. The element of questioning and carrying through on hunches and ideas adds an exciting flavor to day-by-day nursing. Conversely, the researcher may wish to test her concepts in practice. She will also act as consultant and advisor to the nurse who is beginning to collect data and who is interested in objectively studying nursing situations. There is much room for a blending of theory and practice in operating room nursing today.

Fig. 1-4 conceptualizes a framework of nursing theory put forth by Wiedenbach.

> Theory is an abstract phenomenon. It develops within the mind but derives from reality and influences action. It is the outgrowth of an intellectual process set in motion by observations. From them, ideas are generated. Then, by

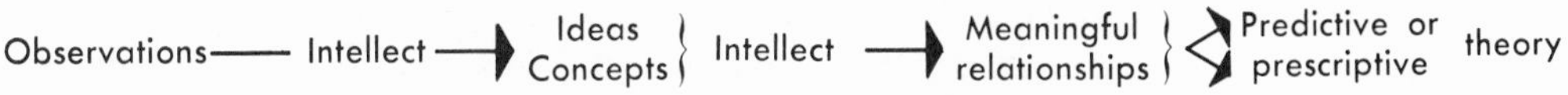

Observations —— Intellect → Ideas Concepts { Intellect → Meaningful relationships { Predictive or prescriptive theory

Fig. 1-4. Nursing theory. (After Wiedenbach.)

means of the intellect, the ideas—we'll call them concepts—may be consciously brought into meaningful relationship with one another for such purposes as to identify or isolate factors, to characterize or classify them, to predict effect from cause, or to prescribe a course of action by which to obtain desired results. When such a relationship is articulated, a theory has been formulated.*

Theory may be viewed as a conceptual foundation or a framework with a purpose. In nursing the purpose of theory is the ultimate application to clinical practice.

A difficulty of analyzing nursing in a theoretical framework comes from the practical application of nursing "the whole person." There is no complete science of the whole human being. Nevertheless, applying some aspects of a discipline is possible, as it is also possible to restructure what is known. For example, caring, as a nursing concept, exists and is specific to the field but has not been made explicit. We do not know exactly how to define "caring" and therefore are unable to completely predict its outcome or use it to full advantage.

Theory-building in operating room nursing need not take place within the confines of a classroom or academic laboratory. It begins with speculation, hunches, impressions, and sometimes even intuition. It is, however, the follow-through of these ideas that transforms them to relevant data. Otherwise the observations may remain only as collected information. If nurses are to practice intelligently, they must alter thinking patterns from mere routine to logical reasoning. Herein lies the answer to wisdom in nursing.

As an example for study, a nurse functioning in the operating room may note an increased incidence in glove punctures and tears. She has a hunch that one brand of surgical gloves may be deficient in manufacturing standards. Thereafter, the nurse begins to keep records of all the brands of gloves used, recording the inadvertent punctures that occur in each glove during surgery. The nurse observes the technics of gloving used by each team member to eliminate variables that would invalidate her data. An example would be one surgeon who gloves incorrectly, placing undue stress on the gloves as he dons them, which possibly causes tearing of the gloves. After the data are refined and accurate objective descriptions obtained, the nurse may then consult a statistician and a nurse researcher in order to collaborate on the findings. Care must be taken, however, to derive meanings and applications only where they truly exist. Thus the assistance of a research expert is recommended at this stage.

---

*Wiedenbach, E.: Nurses' wisdom in nursing theory, Am. J. Nurs. 70(5):1057, May 1970. (Copyright The American Journal of Nursing Company.)

Not only would this nurse have learned the rudiments of data collection, but she would also have refined her observational skills, would have a beginning knowledge of the types of "errors" that may creep into a study, and would have a basic understanding of the possible practical applications. This nurse, then, would have acted on intuition in the beginning but would subsequently have collected information, sought help when needed, and made cautious and careful conclusions about her observations.

Another nurse observes that patients who are scheduled for a particular operative procedure appear more anxious than most. She begins to wonder: Is the anxiety related to the preparation they received? Is there something in Room 4 (to which all of these patients are taken) that is frightening? Is it the response of the nurses in surgery? Is it something about the particular surgeon/anesthesiologist combination? Is it the preoperative medication? Or is it the nature of the symbolism of this particular operation? These are only beginning questions to consider. Some questions cannot be assessed quantitatively. For example, we cannot measure "response of a nurse" unless it is stated in clear, definable terms. This illustration is used only to point up the ways in which a genuine research study may begin. It also characterizes the questioning attitude that is so vital for intelligent nursing care.

Implications for operating room nurse roles are beginning to be found in research. The purpose of one study was to determine if a special nursing intervention with sedated patients awaiting general anesthesia induction in the surgery department would be recalled postoperatively in terms that would indicate facilitation of a positive adaptive response to the stress of impending surgery and the operating room environment. The findings supported the hypothesis that the operating room nurse can facilitate adaptation by focusing on the patient as a person, providing affiliation and preparatory communication, and intervening to help the patient cope with identified adaptation problems.[8]

Much benefit accrues if nurses approach their work with a curious attitude, always seeking to ask "why?" and always searching for better answers and practices. This holds true for the nursing student as well. Even as a beginner the student can make skillful observations, read and study the literature, and constantly refine the concepts of thinking and doing in nursing.

REFERENCES

1. Ethicon suture handbook, Somerville, N.J., 1961, Ethicon, Inc., pp. 1-2.
2. Mandate for the registered nurse as circulator in the operating room; Delegates approve statements, resolutions at twenty-second congress, AORN J. 21:1067-1073, May 1975.
3. Gruendemann, B. J.: Mandate for circulator shows RN role, AORN J. 22:321-322, Sept. 1975.
4. Gruendemann, B. J.: Role of the OR nurse: A literature review, AORN J. 10:57-59, Dec. 1969.
5. Alexander, C., Schrader, E., and Kneedler, J.: Preoperative visits: The OR nurse unmasks, AORN J. 19:401-412, Feb. 1974.

6. Association of Operating Room Nurses and American Nurses' Association Division on Medical-Surgical Nursing Practice: Standards of nursing practice: Operating room, Kansas City, Mo., 1975, American Nurses' Association.
7. Gruendemann, B. J., Hunter, A. R., Kneedler, J. A., and Schick, D.: Nursing audit: Challenge to the operating room nurse, Denver, 1974, Association of Operating Room Nurses.
8. Nolan, M. R.: The effects of nursing intervention in the operating room as recalled on the third postoperative day, Unpublished Master's Thesis, Los Angeles, 1974, University of California.

SUGGESTED READINGS

Abdellah, F. G., and Levine, E.: Better patient care through nursing research, New York, 1971, Macmillan, Inc.
Abdellah, F. G., and others: New directions in patient-centered nursing, New York, 1973, Macmillan, Inc.
Cantlin, V. L.: O.R. nursing is a professional specialty, Nurs. Outlook 8:376-378, July 1960.
Diers, D.: This I believe—about nursing research, Nurs. Outlook 18:50-54, Nov. 1970.
Dodge, G. H.: Nurses reveal a restless attitude towards research, AORN J. 20:747-751, Nov. 1974.
Ellis, R.: The practitioner as theorist, Am. J. Nurs. 69:1434-1438, July 1969.
Hesterly, S. C.: You are the patient's advocate, AORN J. 17:204-209, April 1973.
Jacox, A. K.: The pursuit of excellence as a professional goal, AORN J. 21:1240-1308, June 1975.
Kneedler, J. A.: What is the nurse's part in OR scenario? AORN J. 24:849-852, Nov. 1976.
Lang, N. M.: Quality assurance in nursing, AORN J. 22:18-186, Aug. 1975.
McBride, M. A., Diers, D., and Schmidt, R. L.: Nurse-researcher: The crucial hyphen, Am. J. Nurs. 70:1256-1260, June 1970.
Minckley, B.: Physiologic and psychologic responses of elective surgical patients, Nurs. Res. 23:392-401, Sept.-Oct. 1974.
Nolan, M. G.: Problem solving is research in action, AORN J. 20:225-231, Aug. 1974.
Plourde, C.: The evolution of OR peer review, AORN J. 24:754-762, Oct. 1976.
Roberts, M., Vilinskas, J., and Owens, G.: Technicians or nurses in the OR, Am. J. Nurs. 74:906-907, May 1974.
Wald, F. S., and Leonard, R. C.: Towards development of nursing practice theory, Nurs. Res. 13:309-313, Fall 1964.
Wiedenbach, E.: The helping art of nursing, Am. J. Nurs. 63:54-57, Nov. 1963.
Yokes, J. A.: Nursing standards measure quality of practice, AORN J. 20:1039-1046, Dec. 1974.

CHAPTER 2

THE EXPERIENCE OF SURGERY
patient and nurse

Broad perspectives of surgery, standards and roles, theoretical foundations, history, and research were discussed in Chapter 1. We hope that these discussions help to set the scene for consideration of surgery, the patient, and the nurse.

In this chapter a diagram-model is presented of the patient-nurse interaction throughout the surgical experience. A model is an abstraction of reality that aids explanation and understanding. This model incorporates highlights from the discussion in Chapter 1 and points out the necessity of using broad concepts (theoretical) when considering the patient undergoing surgery and the associated nursing roles and actions. Also placed in perspective in the model are succeeding topics in the book, such as asepsis, nursing care plans, instrumentation, and needs of patients.

Fig. 2-1 represents the process of operating room nursing. The operating room nurse interacts with the patient, becomes familiar with his individual needs and uniqueness, and devises *care* that complements either the process of recovery and adjustment or dying with dignity.

Throughout the patient's entire hospitalization the nurse will have a consistently beneficial effect on the patient's outcome only if two factors are constantly kept in mind: (1) the personal uniqueness of *each* patient, and (2) the common needs and requirements of *all* patients. These two factors are depicted in Fig. 2-1 as "personal, individual considerations" and "general nursing considerations." All operating room nursing care is predicated on these two keypoints to care.

The operating room nurse is primarily the patient's advocate in the process of either remaining or becoming well or of reaching the end of life. The nurse provides vital support and assists the physician in certain aspects of his therapy, but she does much more than carry out physician's orders. The operating room nurse is the change agent—the catalyst—in

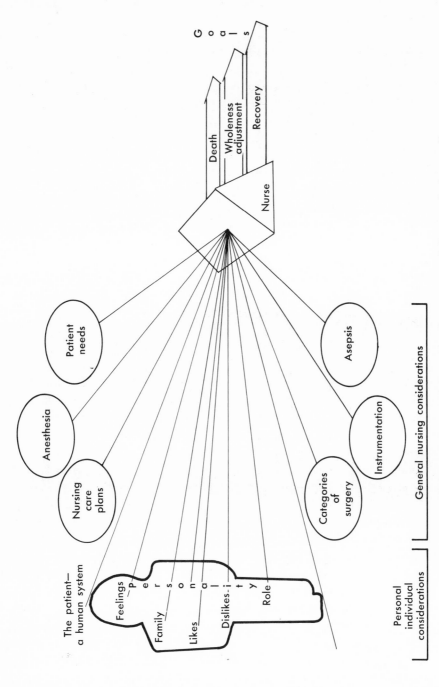

Fig. 2-1. Nurse-patient interaction during the process of the surgical experience.

the processes of convalescence or dying. The nurse is the person who gives *skilled care with concern* and interacts purposefully with the patient. Nursing action should *facilitate* and *enhance* those processes that best meet the patient's needs.

The nurse's interaction with the patient becomes sophisticated when she both understands herself and considers the patient's needs and unique "oneness." Whether the patient is awake and alert on the nursing unit or anesthetized in the operating room, the nurse has a vital role in determining the outcome of the surgical experience.

In Fig. 2-1 nursing action is likened to a focal point of incoming cues, observations, and principles of care. The care that results should serve as a broadening, learning experience for both nurse and patient. Outcomes, recovery or death, must reflect this effort on the part of the nurse. Her knowledge and skill will be used to advantage as she cares for each surgical patient and as she uses herself therapeutically.

THE PERSON AS A PATIENT

Each person is an integrated, complex being—an entity. This person must be visualized as one human organism, not as a body divided into physical, emotional, and spiritual compartments. Although these distinctions are sometimes made, they should be used for *study purposes only*. The person must be considered as one unified whole, with the entire body system functioning as a coordinated unit. (The term "system" is used here in the context of an ordered, unitary whole. Reference is *not* to groups of body tissues and organs with similar functions, such as digestive, respiratory, and circulatory systems. An understanding of this distinction is necessary in order to fully comprehend the meaning of Fig. 2-1.)

This "whole" is more than just a sum of the activities of the various body organs or units. It is an almost mysterious, coordinated set of responses that calls forth appropriate reactions from persons and situations around it. Integrated into a phenomenal complexity, the whole still has an order and organization that allows for both freedom and purpose in its response.

In both research and practice the coordinated interdependence of body and mind is constantly apparent. Levine states, "The absolutes of mind and body are lost in the still-hidden electrochemical pathways of the brain, and the absolutes of the individual and the society are denied by the incessant dependence of one upon the other."*

Studies in the behavioral sciences have demonstrated the importance of more than physical contact in treatment and care of patients. "Personalities" cannot be generalized nor stereotyped, but "behavior" may be consciously guided to effectively serve the needs of patients.

---

*Levine, M. E.: The pursuit of wholeness, Am. J. Nurs. 69(1):94, Jan. 1969. (Copyright The American Journal of Nursing Company.)

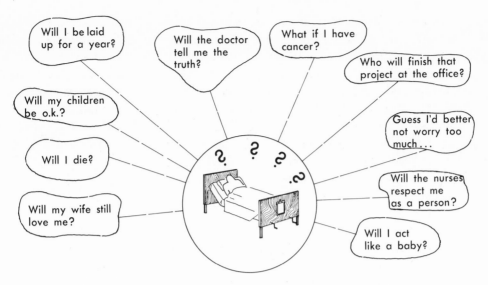

Fig. 2-2. Concerns of the surgical patient.

THE EXPERIENCE OF SURGERY

As the patient arrives in the operating room, his unique approaches and responses are assessed by the operating room nurse. To this patient surgery is one of the most important experiences in his life. It is *his* operation, *his* family, and *his* body. He may seem egocentric, but this should be allowed as he sifts his feelings and thoughts, healthy and unhealthy, into some mode of acting that has meaning to *him*.

Nurses may habitually categorize a patient as "a gallbladder," "a broken leg," or "a T & A," in order to fit him into an efficient frame of reference in terms of *procedure*. They will be more effective, however, if they first evaluate the patient as a *human* who has brought his family, work, environment, and body image—all unique—to the hospital with him (Fig. 2-2). From this springboard the nurse is best able to plan care *with* a patient—care that is personally tailored to fit him.

Surgery, in itself, may present a threat, conscious or subconscious, to the person who must undergo it. If an illness is superimposed on the surgery as another threat, the feelings may become magnified. This is true especially if the illness has been accompanied by stressors such as pain, nausea and vomiting, drainage, or forced immobility. There may also be doubts that surgery will relieve the aggravating symptoms. "Will the operation be successful?" "Will I really feel better after it's over?" "Will my family accept a change in my appearance?"

Regression and dependency are expected accompaniments of surgery. Both the threat of surgery and the hospital environment force an almost childlike, passive behavior on the patient. The nurse must assess the patient's own perceptions of the stress associated with surgery and not interject her own feelings of how she thinks the patient *should* be feeling or acting. It is easy, but erroneous, to assume that the patient scheduled for "minor" surgery will experience less stress than one scheduled for "major" surgery. Surgery is not a neutral event for the patient, and pre-judgments and false assumptions must be avoided. Hospital routines must be followed, but sometimes they ignore the real needs of those they should serve—the patients.

These situations present special and potent opportunities for the operating room nurse. There are at least as many challenges as there are patients if the nurse sincerely accepts the premise that every patient is unique.

The nurse usually sees patients at times when they are suffering personal stress involving crises of varying intensities. Some mechanisms of adjustment and adaptation succeed and some fail. Surgical patients, unlike medical patients, also know they must face a period of possible unconsciousness, pain, discomfort, and stress *before* they reach the convalescent phase. They do not come to the hospital with the expectation of immediate rest and restoration, even if theirs is elective surgery. Skillful nurses use this knowledge in their interaction with patients. They encourage patients to release stored up feelings, if they so desire. They actively listen, without interjecting their own opinions of how the patient should think and act. They create an atmosphere in which each person feels free to express himself without being belittled. The nurse instills confidence with calm explanations coupled with technical skills. These principles, incorporated into the care given, will aid the patient and his family in approaching surgery with as little harmful distress as possible.

Anxiety is present in most patients about to undergo surgery. It may be apparent in crying or constant restless activity; often however, it is covert, or concealed. The patient may appear calm and composed to the nurse when in reality he feels helpless and panic-stricken.

The operating room nurse should recognize that anxiety is both *common and normal* in surgical patients and should reassure patients of this fact. The nurse can do much to alleviate or manage the distress associated with anxiety, even though the anxiety itself is not dissipated. Patients may or may not wish to talk about their feelings. In many cases the causes of anxiety are unconscious and cannot be verbalized, no matter how aggravating. All the patient may be able to recognize is that he is "mighty scared," "nervous," or "jittery." The sensitive nurse does not pry, but accepts the patient along with his feelings and his *peculiar expressions of* these feelings. Verbal and nonverbal communication of acceptance must be conveyed to the patient.

How each patient feels about his surgery depends a great deal on the specific body part involved. Is it socially acceptable to speak of the type of operation he is to have? Will his relatives consider his "uncleanliness" to have led to a need for the surgery? Is the body part involved in sexual functions or reproduction? Will the operation change the appearance of his face and hands? A person's body image may be greatly affected by the surgical procedure, whether it is labeled "major" or "minor." The nurse considers this in her initial assessment of the patient.[1]

The body organ involved may be a known and unknown seat of symbolism, hostility, resentment, or enjoyment. Psychosomatic symptoms and altered body responses that have been well established over the years and used as "crutches" may be alleviated by the surgery, to either the disgust or delight of the patient. A hallowed body condition, such as a "nervous stomach," even though physically unhealthy, may have been the source of equilibrium for the patient. In this case surgery may be seen by the patient as more of a threat to his equilibrium than as a means of relief from troublesome or annoying symptoms. As stated by Larsen:

> To those patients who have managed to control others with their "gall-bladder attacks" or their "stomach trouble," the loss of this secret weapon through surgery will mean loss of personal power and prestige. To others, removal of a focus of resented pain may open a new chapter of enjoyment and life activity.*

Other feelings of the patient frequently encountered by the operating room nurse include ambivalence, guilt, embarrassment, bewilderment, panic, anger, and fear of known or unknown dangers. Fear of losing control or of being unaware of one's surroundings is very real and frightening to many patients. Some persons fear anesthesia (being unaware) much more than the scalpel or the surgery itself.

Occasionally overlooked and disregarded is the patient who comes to the hospital with a sense of welcome relief. Having had to cope with very debilitating symptoms, such as acute gallbladder spasms, this patient is *happy to be in the hospital* even though he is anxious to some degree. He is grateful that he will soon be relieved of his aggravating symptoms. The nurse's understanding of these feelings is just as vital as her understanding of patterns of hostility or anger.

PRINCIPLES OF NURSING ACTION

As shown in Fig. 2-1, the care that the operating room nurse gives may be viewed as a point of focus. If the care is skilled and effective, the results may provide a positive learning experience for the patient and the nurse. However, if the nurse fails to use herself and her nursing knowledge effectively, the result may be narrow and limited, culminating in a dissatisfied patient. The patient may have a stormy course of recovery, or he may be unable to resolve the anxiety experienced during hospitalization. The nurse's judgment and *caring* ability may determine the effect of her action.

Ideally, the nurse is a catalyst in the induction of a favorable response

---

*Larsen, V. L.: What hospitalization means to patients, Am. J. Nurs. **61**:(5):47, May 1961. (Copyright The American Journal of Nursing Company.)

by the patient to his surgical experience. In this role the nurse assists and complements the patient in activities he is unable to do for himself.

Ministering to the surgical patient requires a working knowledge of his individuality—assessment of the "real person." But it also requires working knowledge of additional nursing skills, which are probably more easily taught, defined, and transferred from one situation to another. Fig. 2-1 shows certain nursing skills labeled "general nursing considerations." These are the constants in nursing care—the considerations every patient must receive if his care is to be effective. Nursing care, whether in or out of the operating suite, must include knowledge and exact application of the principles of asepsis. In addition the application of the nursing process (including the use of nursing care plans) serves as a vital link in the continuity of care chain. If the nurse does not have a systematic approach in dealing with her patients, care is haphazard, sporadic, and done under trial and error conditions.

To effectively fulfill their role in the operating room, nurses must have basic knowledge of anesthesia technics and agents; they should also be thoroughly familiar with instrumentation. ("Instrumentation" does not refer to rote memory of all instruments used, but rather to an understanding of groups of instruments by virtue of their usage in different types of surgery.) Preoperative and postoperative interviews are indispensable in the care of the surgical patient and provide another link in the chain of continuity.

The preceding topics are all considered in depth in succeeding chapters. Important aspects of recovery room care are also considered.

Other nursing considerations are included in Fig. 2-1 because they are a part of the fundamentals of operating room nursing action. One of these is *needs* of patients. In daily hospital situations there are common patient requirements, which help determine care. These identified needs are standard factors to most nurses but are frequently overlooked as determinants of nursing care.

It may safely be assumed that all patients, because they are humans, have certain needs and wants. The predominance of one particular need and the priorities, balance, and distribution of patients' needs will differ. The type of surgery will also affect the needs or functional requirements. Nursing care must be planned around human needs.

The human body has a basic requirement for *activity, rest, and sleep. Safety and protection* refer to environmental conditions and include physical safety in the hospital as well as in the home. Other essential requirements are those for *nutrition* of all body cells, *regulation* of body processes (especially neural and chemical), *oxygen-carbon dioxide exchange,* and *elimination* of wastes and excess body products.

Each person has a basic need for *interpersonal relationships,* which may include the concept of the presence of higher beings (sometimes termed *spiritual* needs). Verbal and nonverbal *communications* may be seen as a part of the person's interaction with his surroundings.

The needs approach is useful particularly in determining necessary action by the operating room nurse. Because this approach is discussed at length in most nursing fundamentals and medical-surgical texts, the subject will not be elaborated upon here. The reader is directed to Abdellah's work[2] on needs and related nursing problems.

Another model of nursing, the Roy Adaptation Model, is helpful in conceptualizing operating room nursing. In this model the nurse focuses on the patient as a biopsychosocial being who is constantly interacting with his changing internal and external environment. Needs of the patient are for physiologic, psychosocial, and affiliational integrity. Detailed explanations and assessment tools are available and can be applied to surgical patients.[3]

CATEGORIES OF SURGERY

Surgical operative procedures have traditionally been classified in groups according to the body parts or physical systems involved or according to the surgical specialties. Examples are: abdominal, thoracic, orthopedic, plastic, and urologic surgery. These broad headings are functional for both the surgeon and the person who prepares the instruments and equipment for each procedure.

These time-honored groupings of surgery are not purposeful for the operating room nurse who plans her care around the individual, because they fail to account for the *person* who is to undergo the surgery. They cannot be used as the foremost criteria for planning nursing care. Neither are these classifications helpful to nursing students as they learn to fit preoperative and postoperative care to the patient's needs.

That classifications are necessary is not disputed. Categories are needed that (1) reflect the patient's individuality; (2) stimulate all nurses, students and graduates alike, to always question procedures and the reasons for surgery; (3) consider commonalities, such as instrumentation, asepsis, and anesthesia principles as inherent, contributing components; and (4) require a knowledge of the exact surgical procedure performed.

A suggested approach to divisions of surgery consists of the following six categories:
1. Surgery involving loss of body part, organ, or function
2. Surgery involving the removal of a tumor, cyst, or foreign body
3. Surgery for diagnosis
4. Surgery for the insertion, removal, or application of a prosthesis, graft, transplant, or therapeutic device
5. Surgery for reconstruction
6. Surgery to establish drainage or reestablish a passageway

As guides for study and criteria for devising nursing care plans, these divisions are useful to nursing students during their operating room nursing experience. In this conceptual scheme the student evaluates the surgical patients, their surgical treatment, and the diagnoses and background history. Surgery is seen in a broader perspective than that of the procedure alone.

A discussion of each of the six divisions will include examples of types of patients and procedures that may be included and nursing problems that may be anticipated in each category. It must be emphasized that the procedural examples are only that. Certain surgeries, such as gastric resection, may be done for one of several reasons and thus fit into more than one of the six categories. Therefore, detailed knowledge of each patient is necessary before placement on this list. The procedural examples are not intended to be all-inclusive; the reader is urged to make additions to the lists from his own experiences.

1. Surgery involving loss of body part, organ, or function

Procedural examples: cholecystectomy, appendectomy, gastric resection, abdominal-perineal resection, hysterectomy, amputation, orchiectomy, cataract extraction, lobectomy, prostatectomy, tonsillectomy and adenoidectomy, cast application, thyroidectomy, mastectomy, nephrectomy, vein stripping, sympathectomy, vagotomy, laminectomy, vasectomy, splenectomy, excision of ganglion

Loss of a body part may have wide-ranging consequences for the patient. If the organ or part has been the seat of much symbolism for the patient, a long period of readjustment may be anticipated as in patients undergoing hysterectomies, mastectomies, prostatectomies, and orchiectomies. A change in body function or appearance may be a major threat to these patients. Physiologic disturbances, such as hormone imbalance, may also result.

Reestablishing function for an amputee presents a challenging nursing problem. Patients having cast applications must be assisted to accept a temporary loss of function and incapacitation. Finding diversional activities may be a primary nursing action.

After cataract extractions the patient cannot see for a period of time. Skilled care to assure safety and security must be provided.

If the body part has been diseased and the cause of much distress, the loss may be welcomed by the patient. For example, if the saphenous vein has become unsightly and the cause for comments and embarrassment, the patient usually looks forward to its removal. Acceptance by friends and family members may be a key motivating force for removal of a body part or organ.

2. Surgery involving the removal of a tumor, cyst, or foreign body

Procedural examples: prostate gland resection, cyst and mole removals, lithotomy, ureterolithotomy, pyelolithotomy, parotid tumor excision, branchial cyst excision, ovarian cystectomy, embolectomy, pilonidal cystectomy, litholapaxy, and those from category 1, if a tumor was present

Nursing care of this group of patients may be quite similar to that of the patient in category 1, depending on whether removal of an abnormal growth also involves the excision of the entire body part or organ in which it is located. An ovarian cystectomy may mean the excision of the cyst alone or the removal of the cyst and the ovary. Removal of foreign bodies, such as calculi, may also be accompanied by excision of the body part.

To recognize these fine points of surgery is also to recognize and anticipate physiologic changes and possible compensations of one body organ for another.

Of particular importance in this group of patients is the nature of the neoplasm excised. If the patient is prepared to accept the diagnosis of malignancy, will the final reality be too much to accept? Is there metastasis of the original tumor? Exactly what information has the patient been given and what is he capable of accepting? On the other hand, a diagnosis of benign tumor almost always brings welcome relief.

The nurse must be prepared to listen and encourage thoughts about the diagnosis, reactions, and accompanying frustrations.

---

3. Surgery for diagnosis
Procedural examples: explorations, biopsies, dilatation and curettage of the cervix and uterus, pneumoencephalogram, myelogram, cystoscopy, bronchoscopy, esophagoscopy, laryngoscopy, proctoscopy, laparoscopy, mediastinoscopy, hysterosalpingogram, culdoscopy, arthroscopy

---

Because this patient undergoes agonizing periods of anticipation and repressed guilt and anger, supportive nursing care is a priority in category 3. Keeping communication lines open can make a taxing period at least tolerable. The patient and his family must know that the nurse is available to them. The nurse must also convey genuine understanding during a period that may be very trying and must be prepared to answer the many questions this patient may have. "When will I know the outcome?" "What if I need more surgery?" "Do other people go through the same feelings?" "Do you think everything will turn out OK?"

---

4. Surgery for the insertion, removal, or application of a prosthesis, graft, transplant, or therapeutic device
Procedural examples: insertion of hip prosthesis, vein graft, arterial graft, heart transplant, kidney transplant, skin graft, Shea procedure, radium insertion, hip nailing, insertion of Kirschner wires, bone grafts, total hip replacement, removal of nail or pin, joint replacements

---

Maintenance of good body alignment and function and the prevention of contractures and other deformities may be anticipated as nursing problems in this division of surgery.

Adjustment in both attitude and function to a body replacement or prosthesis will require much effort and work by the patient. Nursing care that includes encouragement and teaching will be the most effective and helpful.

In this era of transplants the nurse must also consider ethical and moral implications of surgery that involves human body part replacement. Deep-seated, intense reactions may be expected from the recipient and the families of both the donor and recipient.

Changes in appearance may result from grafting procedures. Sensitivity to these changes must be recognized by the nurse and treated in an accepting and realistic manner.

---

5. Surgery for reconstruction

Procedural examples: tendon repairs, tympanoplasty, colporrhaphy, arthrotomy, herniorrhaphy, trachelorrhaphy, hysteropexy, orchiopexy, Shirodkar procedure, circumcision, cleft lip and palate repairs, spinal fusions, submucous resection, burn debridement, fracture reduction, eye muscle repair, cranioplasty, cervical cauterization, rhytidectomy

---

Reconstructive surgery may fulfill a person's desire for better appearance, increased function, and a greater degree of happiness. It may represent an anticipated period of discomfort with questionable results. Even with the best of hopes, this type of surgery may fail to produce the desired outcome.

Repeated operations may be necessary for certain patients, such as those with recurrent hernias or those with middle ear conditions requiring several tympanoplasties. Immobility may be a result of surgery such as fracture reductions.

A school-aged child may be highly embarrassed by having to undergo a circumcision or surgery for undescended testicles. The considerate nurse will understand this and similar patient reactions and assist appropriately in the rehabilitation process.

---

6. Surgery to establish drainage or reestablish a passageway

Procedural examples: nephrostomy, cystostomy, tracheostomy, gastrostomy, antrostomy, fenestration, incision and drainage of abscess, myringotomy, thoracotomy, Caldwell-Luc procedure, repair of pyloric stenosis, ureterolithotomy, colostomy, ileostomy

---

Almost every patient who undergoes this type of surgery will have drainage and drainage catheters or devices. A prime nursing function is the maintenance of scrupulous cleanliness and the provision for tube or orifice patency and drainage. Odors may be present, especially if there is purulent drainage. Prevention of infection is a high nursing priority.

Preparation for this type of surgery might include reinforcement of the surgeon's explanations and clarification of the use of tubes and expected drainage, including care of catheters.

When functions will be altered, a careful explanation with ample opportunity for feedback and questions from the patient must be included preoperatively.

POSTSURGERY OUTCOMES

The outcome of the patient's surgery is, to a great extent, dependent on the skill and technics of the surgeon. It also depends on the condition of the patient, the preoperative diagnosis, the extent of the disease or malfunction, and the environment in which surgery took place.

The skills of the nurse in the operating room will have an influence on the patient's outcome. Nursing skills also affect the ability of the surgeon to perform the surgery and therefore affect the patient's outcome in an indirect way. The operating room nurse plays a vital role in preparing and maintaining an exact, optimal environment for the performance of surgery.

Postoperative nursing care does make a difference in the recovery of a patient. Polished nursing technics, such as the changing of dressings or irrigation of catheters, affect the rate and quality of wound healing. Attention to ambulation and nutritional needs influences the body's return to normalcy. The nurse's attitudes and understanding, reflected in words and actions, are powerful forces in the attainment of comfort and rapid recovery.

The nurse must assist some patients in planning for and adjusting to an extended period of convalescence. Families must be included throughout the entire phase. If the patient does not or will not recover, the utmost in dignity and respect must be given when death is approaching or ensues.

Readjustment to a new way of life after surgery may be necessary. Adaptation may be difficult and may require much work and effort on the part of the patient. Every patient depends on the nurse for guidance during this period.

REFERENCES

1. Gruendemann, B. J.: The impact of surgery on body image, Nurs. Clin. North Am. 10(4):635-643, Dec. 1975.
2. Abdellah, F. G., and others: Patient-centered approaches to nursing, New York, 1960, Macmillan, Inc.
3. Roy, Sister Callista: Introduction to nursing: An adaptation model, Englewood Cliffs, N.J., 1976, Prentice-Hall, Inc.

SUGGESTED READINGS

Aasterud, M.: Defenses against anxiety in the nurse-patient relationship, Nurs. Forum 1:35-59, Summer 1962.
Barnett, L. A.: Preparing your patient for the operating room, AORN J. 18:534-539, Sept. 1973.
Engel, G. L.: Grief and grieving, Am. J. Nurs. 64:95-98, Sept. 1964.
Field, L. W.: Identifying the psychological aspects of the surgical patient, AORN J. 17:86-90, Jan. 1973.
Graham, L. E., and Conley, E. M.: Evaluation of anxiety and fear in adult surgical patients, Nurs. Res. 20:113-122, March-April 1971.
Howells, J. G., editor: Modern perspectives in the psychiatric aspects of surgery, New York, 1976, Brunner/Mazel, Inc.
Janis, I. L.: Psychological stress: Psychoanalytical and behavioral studies of surgical patients, New York, 1958, John Wiley & Sons, Inc.
Janis, I. L.: Stress and frustration, New York, 1971, Harcourt Brace Jovanovich, Inc.
Johnson, J. E., Dabbs, J. M., Jr., and Levanthal, H.: Psychosocial factors in the welfare of surgical patients, Nurs. Res. 19:18-29, Jan.-Feb. 1970.

Levine, M. E.: Adaptation and assessment—A rationale for nursing intervention, Am. J. Nurs. 66:2450-2453, Nov. 1966.

Levine, M. E.: Holistic nursing, Nurs. Clin. North Am. 6(2):253-264, June 1971.

Norris, C. M.: The professional nurse and body image. In Carolyn E. Carlson, coordinator: Behavioral concepts and nursing intervention, Philadelphia, 1970, J. B. Lippincott Co., pp. 39-65.

Norris, C. M.: The work of getting well, Am. J. Nurs. 69:2118-2121, Oct. 1969.

Piepgras, R.: The other dimension: Spiritual help, Am. J. Nurs. 68:2610-2613, Dec. 1968.

Pleitez, J. A.: Psychological complications of the surgical patient, AORN J. 16:137-146, Aug. 1972.

Ring, W. H.: Child vs. adult: The OR patient's personality, AORN J. 16:101-106, Sept. 1972.

Rosenthal, S.: Stress in the surgical patient: A review, New Physician 13:308-310, Sept. 1964.

Rubin, R.: Body image and self esteem, Nurs. Outlook 16:20-23, June 1968.

Saylor, D. E.: Understanding presurgical anxiety, AORN J. 22:624-636, Oct. 1975.

Symposium on the concept of body image, R. Murray, guest editor, Nurs. Clin. North Am. 7(4):593-707, Dec. 1972.

Titchener, J. L., and Levine, M.: Surgery as a human experience, New York, 1960, Oxford University Press, Inc.

Trail, I. D., and Monke, J. V.: Psychic sequelae of surgical change in body structure, Nurs. Forum 2:14-23, 1963.

Wells, R. W.: Body image and surgical alterations, AORN J. 21:812-815, April 1975.

Wolfer, J. A., and Davis, C. E.: Assessment of surgical patient's preoperative emotional condition and postoperative welfare, Nurs. Res. 19:402-414, Sept.-Oct. 1970.

CHAPTER 3

LEGAL AND ETHICAL IMPLICATIONS

CONTINUITY AND TEAMWORK

A team is a group of people working toward a common goal. The health team is that group of persons concerned with the health needs of a particular patient. Although each individual has appointed functions, the team concept supports overlapping of functions to achieve the common goal. Shared functions have particular legal and ethical implications.

In the past one physician assisted by one nurse represented the health care team. The team of today, however, has many members because of both technical and social advances. The result of the original concepts of team nursing was a tendency for the registered nurse to be moved away from the patient's side and into the role of care *director* rather than care *deliverer*. Recent trends, however, that involve the patient as a *participant* on the team with prerogatives as to when, where, and how his care will occur have aided in returning the nurse to the patient.

In addition, health team responsibilities have evolved so that individual members now function less in a highly subordinate relationship and more as colleagues, with functions moving from one team member to another in keeping with changing demands. With the surgeon understandably focusing on procedures and technics and the anesthesiologist involved with physiologic modalities, the operating room nurse assumes responsibility for the patient's safety and progress during the surgical experience. Implicit to accepting this responsibility is the nurse's commitment to advocacy in behalf of the patient based on her nursing knowledge of the patient's needs. It is the appropriate role of the nurse to maintain the individuality of the patient as a person and to assist in maintaining a safe, therapeutic environment for the patient, physically and psychologically. This is important because the smoother the course of the procedure, the less tension for the team members, and the better the result for the patient.

Operating room nurses must also accept the challenge to become vital *nursing team* members to enhance the continuity of patient care. To achieve

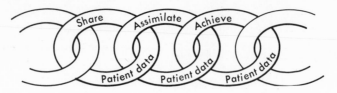

Fig. 3-1. Continuity of patient care.

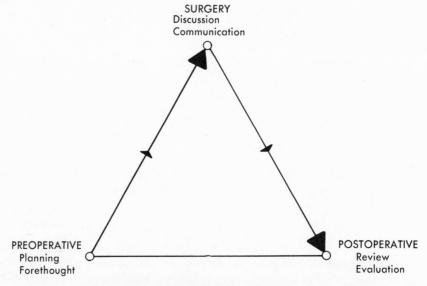

Fig. 3-2. Surgical continuity.

continuity, there must be communication. Continuity also implies that accurate information about the patient accompanies him to any unit of the hospital. To gain continuity, the team members must communicate, listen, share, interpret, and act in behalf of the surgical patient. A continuous chain of care requires that patient data must first be *shared,* second *assimilated,* and third *achieved* (Fig. 3-1). Each link in the chain is essential to the final outcome. The operating room nurse has unparalleled opportunities to provide therapeutic direction to this chain of care.

Continuity can also be used to describe the ideal surgical experience. The ideal to be achieved is an unbroken, coherent whole reflecting a continuous high quality of care. The best and easiest way to achieve this quality is by (1) *planning and forethought,* (2) *discussion and communication,* and (3) *review and evaluation* (Fig. 3-2). Surgery may be the critical point in the patient's hospitalization; effective preoperative care is calculated to provide for every eventuality of this crucial event, and definitive postoperative care emanates from it.

By using the team approach the team members will evolve a care plan that will reflect their planning and forethought. The nurse fulfills the criteria of discussion and communication by conscientiously recording the events occurring during the surgical procedure and supplementing these records when indicated so that those involved in postoperative care will be aware of the chain of events occurring during surgery. Review and evaluation are accomplished by seeing the patient as often as possible postoperatively in order to assess the nursing care plan and to determine the degree of success achieved in meeting the prescribed goals.

A basic understanding of the laws that govern the practice of nursing and certain ethical issues that influence this practice is necessary to enable the nurse to assume her proper place on the health care team.

NURSING PRACTICE ACTS

Part of the difficulty that occurs when attempting to discuss the legalities of nursing practice is that the definition of nursing is still evolving. Many and varied approaches have been used, resulting in revised nurse practice acts in many states. The California Nurse Practice Act is offered as an example of one that provides for the future. It should be noted that care was exercised to avoid itemizing *procedures* since it was believed that "laundry-list" laws are delimiting.

> AB 3124: Section 1. Section 2725
> In amending this section at the 1973-74 session, the Legislature recognizes that nursing is a dynamic field, the practice of which is continually evolving to include more sophisticated patient care activities. It is the intent of the Legislature to provide clear legal authority for functions and procedures which have common acceptance and usage. It is the legislative intent also to recognize the existence of overlapping functions between physicians and registered nurses and to permit additional sharing of functions within organized health care systems which provide for collaboration between physicians and registered nurses.
>
> The practice of nursing within the meaning of this chapter means those functions helping people cope with difficulties in daily living which are associated with their actual or potential health or illness problems or the treatment hereof which require a substantial amount of scientific knowledge or technical skill, and includes all of the following:
>
> a. Direct and indirect patient care services that insure the safety, comfort, personal hygiene, and protection of patients; and the performance of disease prevention and restoration measures.
>
> b. Direct and indirect patient care services, including but not limited to, the administration of medications and therapeutic agents, necessary to implement a treatment, disease prevention, or rehabilitative regimen prescribed by a physician, dentist or podiatrist.
>
> c. The performance of basic health care, testing, and prevention procedures, including, but not limited to, skin tests, immunization techniques, and the withdrawal of human blood from veins and arteries.
>
> d. Observation of signs and symptoms of illness, reactions to treatment, general behavior, or general physical condition, and (1) determination of whether such signs, symptoms, reactions, behavior or general appearance exhibit abnormal characteristics; and (2) implementation, based on observed abnormalities, of appropriate reporting, or referral, or standardized procedures, or changes in treatment regimen in accordance with standardized procedures, or the initiation of emergency procedures. "Standardized procedures" as used in this section means policies or protocols developed for an organized health care system through collaboration among administrators and health professionals including physicians and nurses.

Historically, much of what was once considered the practice of medicine has become part of the practice of nursing. This shift has occurred because the hospital is increasingly being used as the main base of episodic health care, and it is the nurse who is present when the crisis occurs. The minute saved by having a trained practitioner present who can take definitive action may well be the minute that makes the difference between life and death.

Laws such as California's attempt to protect the nurse in the new areas of function. Further, they serve to encourage nurses to expand their own roles in practice. Finally, these laws are a mandate to the individual nurse to maintain her competency and skill level.

Another way in which nurses are provided with information relevant to their area of practice is through the efforts of the state nursing associations. Committees have long been at work providing suggestions on safe practice or guidelines for practice.

ROLE CHANGES

In the days of the "captain of the ship" concept, it was assumed that the physician was totally responsible and liable for all acts relating to patient care. Now, however, we know and recognize that *each individual* is *legally liable* for his own acts; *responsibility* often becomes merely an ethical concern. This has resulted from the increasing complexity of surgical practice with a corresponding need for increased skills, numbers of health team members, and a high level of public awareness and sophistication.

"The picture of the devoted nurse providing humanitarian services for her patient, oblivious to the rest of the world around her, has faded, if in fact it ever did exist, except in the minds of folk hero creators."* The humanitarian or *ethical* aspects of nursing practice are now associated with the *legal* aspects of practice, and the modern nurse must function in a manner appropriately modified by this new area of personal liability.

Every registered nurse should have malpractice insurance coverage. Information about a variety of insurance plans may be obtained through the American Nurses' Association, state nursing associations, or specialty nursing organizations. Although most employing agencies have insurance that provides coverage for acts of the nurse while on duty, those policies represent the interest of the agency and not necessarily those of the nurse.

INFORMED CONSENT

The courts have upheld the right of the patient to be informed of the nature of the treatment, the risk and complications, together with alternative forms of treatment while further stipulating that the responsibility

---

*Sarner, H.: The nurse and the law, Philadelphia, 1968, W. B. Saunders Co., p. iii. (Reprinted with permission.)

for ensuring this right lies with the physician. However, the courts have also stated that the hospital (or its agent) should assure itself that the physician has fulfilled this obligation. To this end, the signature of the patient or his valid representative is obtained on a consent form during the course of hospital care. In many hospitals the nurse frequently is the individual to whom the task of obtaining the signature on surgical consents is delegated. It is the responsibility of the hospital to provide a policy or procedure whereby the nurse, if she believes the patient lacks information, has a method with which to protect both the patient's right and herself from unjustified criticism.

THE "REASONABLE MAN" DOCTRINE

One of the most important criteria by which nurses should view their practice is in terms of what constitutes negligence and what constitutes malpractice. *Negligence* is defined as a failure to exercise the care that a reasonable, prudent person usually exercises. *Malpractice* is misconduct or improper practice in any professional position. It is the duty of the nurse to practice nursing in such a fashion that the standards of the *reasonable man* doctrine are met. The courts have stated that the nurse must act like a reasonably prudent nurse.[1]

The nurse has the responsibility to follow orders or *not* to follow orders lest she find herself legally liable. If the orders under which the nurse functions would not be questioned by a reasonably prudent nurse, there can be no personal liability. If, however, the nurse carries out an order that would cause question in the mind of the reasonably prudent nurse, the nurse is then personally liable.

Nurses are liable for their own negligent conduct. In a California court decision, both the hospital and the doctor were found *not* guilty of negligence or malpractice when the doctor administered formalin instead of novacaine. The nurse had provided the doctor with the wrong agent. The court stated that the physician was entitled to rely on the nurse to properly provide drugs, medicines, and instruments without personally checking them.[2]

Items "lost" during an operation present complex problems of determining where the negligence lies. Current decisions have been against both the nurse and the physician.[3] The nurse was held liable for reporting the sponge count as correct when the subsequent findings proved it incorrect. The physician was found liable for not examining the wound to ascertain, for himself, the number of sponges.[4] It has been said that counts in the operating room are an abomination necessitated by the public's sensitivity to litigation. *What* is counted and *when* it is counted have a wide individual variance from hospital to hospital. It would be philosophical to debate in this forum what, when, and how. However, it is the belief of the authors of this text that counts are done in behalf of the patient to ensure his safety and well-being and should be performed in an organized, systematic manner. It is the responsibility of the hospital to provide policy in support of the counts it authorizes as well as policy for dealing with incorrect counts.

THE "RESPONDEAT SUPERIOR" DOCTRINE

Another major doctrine affecting nursing practice is that of *respondeat superior*. This doctrine states that an employer is legally liable for his employee's negligent conduct that occurs in the furtherance of the employment relationship. Since the patient will undoubtedly bring suit against the nurse's employer because the employer obviously has greater funds, this doctrine offers some measure of protection for the nurse. However, this does not mean that the nurse can act in a rash and hazardous manner in the care of patients. The nurse is also cautioned against a false sense of security. There are court decisions in which the physician and hospital have escaped liability and the nurse has been left to defend the case alone.[5]

The preceding doctrines are the major ones affecting nursing practice. The operating room nurse should also be aware of the important areas of the codes relevant to assault and battery, fraud and deceit, libel and slander, and the invasion of privacy.

RECOMMENDATIONS THAT PROTECT THE PRACTITIONER

The Joint Commission on Accreditation of Hospitals recommends that hospitals provide a written job description for their employees. This would provide the nurse with limits that the hospital imposes on nursing practices. It is further recommended that written policies be provided to the nurse concerning unusual situations that may arise. The hospital is further directed to have on each nursing unit a procedure manual that describes technical functions and the accepted methods of performing these acts.

In the operating room it is advisable to have a supplementary policy/procedure manual that describes rules and regulations of the hospital and the methods of performing technical procedures peculiar to the department. It is suggested that the following data be included: job descriptions for scrub nurse and circulating nurse; personnel and patient scrub and prep routines; cleaning policies; culture procedures; procedures for sponge, instrument, and needle counts; procedure for incorrect counts; chain of command information; information to cover special situations such as cardiac arrest, deaths in the operating room, admission of outside personnel to the operating room, and any others that apply to the facility.

ETHICAL ISSUES

Ethical standards for the nurse were established by the American Nurses' Association in 1950 and revised in 1960, 1968, and 1976. This set of standards is titled "The Code for Nurses with Interpretive Statements."

Adoption of the Code indicates that nurses recognize and accept the responsibilities of their practice and the trust being placed in them. The

Code is a basis for the practice of operating room nursing. The statements of the Code are as follows:

1. The nurse provides services with respect for human dignity and the uniqueness of the client unrestricted by considerations of social or economic status, personal attributes, or the nature of health problems.
2. The nurse safeguards the client's right to privacy by judiciously protecting information of a confidential nature.
3. The nurse acts to safeguard the client and the public when health care and safety are affected by the incompetent, unethical, or illegal practice of any person.
4. The nurse assumes responsibility and accountability for individual nursing judgments and actions.
5. The nurse maintains competence in nursing.
6. The nurse exercises informed judgment and uses individual competence and qualifications as criteria in seeking consultation, accepting responsibilities, and delegating nursing activities to others.
7. The nurse participates in activities that contribute to the ongoing development of the profession's body of knowledge.
8. The nurse participates in the profession's efforts to implement and improve standards of nursing.
9. The nurse participates in the profession's efforts to establish and maintain conditions of employment conducive to high quality nursing care.
10. The nurse participates in the profession's effort to protect the public from misinformation and misrepresentation and to maintain the integrity of nursing.
11. The nurse collaborates with members of the health professions and other citizens in promoting community and national efforts to meet the health needs of the public.*

Membership in professional organizations is voluntary, but necessary. This, together with adherence to the tenets of the Code, is essential to the professionalism of the operating room nurse.

---

*Reprinted with permission from the American Nurses' Association.

REFERENCES
1. Leonard v. Watsonville Community Hospital, 291 P. 2d 496, California, 1956.
2. Hallinan v. Prindle, 62 P. 2d 1075, California, 1937.
3. Piper v. Epstein, 62 N.E. 2d 139, Illinois, 1945.
4. Piper v. Epstein, *supra*.
5. Wood v. Miller, 76 P. 2d 962, Oregon, 1938.

SUGGESTED READINGS
Anderson, D. M., and Cosgriff, J. H.: Partners in practice, Sup. Nurse 5:8-10; 15-16, July 1974.
Bates, B., and Kern, M. S.: Doctor-nurse teamwork: What helps: What hinders? Am. J. Nurs. 67:2066-2071, Oct. 1967.
Berkowitz, N. H., and Malone, M. F.: Intraprofessional conflict, Nurs. Forum 7:50-71, 1968.
Boname, J. R.: Changing attitudes create health care dilemma, AORN J. 22:543-548, Oct. 1975.
Breckenridge, F. J.: Pertinent communication between O.R. and nursing units, Hosp. Topics 43:115-119, June 1965.
Cazalas, M. W.: Legalities and nursing, AORN J. 13:79-86, May 1971.

Creighton, H.: Legal aspects of OR nursing, AORN J. 7:70-74, June 1968.

Crooks, L. C.: Are nurses abdicating their obligations? AORN J. 22:523-529, Oct. 1975.

Dinsmore, R. J.: OR nurse's liability in needle counts, AORN J. 20:1002-1004, Dec. 1974.

Gouge, R. L.: OR nurses face potential liabilities, AORN J. 20:660-665, Oct. 1974.

Hammond, M. J.: Theological implications of organ transplants, AORN J. 9:53-56, March 1969.

Hershey, N.: An expanded role for operating room nurses, AORN J. 18:511-515, Sept. 1973.

Kelly, L. Y.: Nursing practice acts, Am. J. Nurs. 74:1310-1319, July 1974.

Kelly, L. Y.: The patient's right to know, Nurs. Outlook 24:26-32, Jan. 1976.

Lipman, M.: Joint statements—your legal safeguard, RN, pp. 40-44, 69, April 1971.

Ludwig, D.: Winners and losers on the OR team, AORN J. 20:116-128, July 1974.

Lynaugh, J. E., and Bates, B.: The two languages of nursing and medicine, Am. J. Nurs. 73:66-69, Jan. 1973.

Organ, C. H.: OR nurse, surgeon: Common areas of concern, AORN J. 22:898-902, Dec. 1975.

Peeples, E. H., and Francis, G. M.: Social-psychological obstacles to effective health team practice, Nurs. Forum 8:28-37, 1968.

Regan, W. A.: Legally hazardous areas of O.R. nursing, RN 32:86-96, May 1969.

Walker, M. L., and Kasmarik, P. E.: Continuity of care in cardiac surgery, AORN J. 9:62-68, Feb. 1969.

Wilson, R. N.: Teamwork in the operating room. In Jaco, E. G., editor: Patients, physicians and illness, Glencoe, Ill., 1958, The Free Press.

CHAPTER 4

PLANNING SURGICAL PATIENT CARE

"Ever since nursing was first performed, the nurse, by a process either wholly or partially conscious, looked at the patient and determined on the basis of intuition, experience, rote learning, knowledge, or in some cases ignorance, which nursing acts were necessary to relieve his distress."* Obviously, this method left much to the individual nurse practitioner's own sense of commitment (or lack of) to *plan* for her patient. Some patients received planned care; some did not. Thought was sometimes given to the *priority* of patient needs, but usually rote learning was employed. As a result, time was frequently expended meeting needs that the nurse thought the patient *ought* to have, whether he did or not. How often have you heard the not-so-funny story about the patient being awakened to be administered a sleeping pill? Or the one about being sent to the hospital for a rest only to be awakened at 5 AM for a temperature check?

Sadly, it was the things that nurses did wrong that provoked conscientious nurses the nation over to begin a search for better methods of meeting patient care needs. From the desire to find a better method rose the evident need for better *tools* to identify patient needs. If needs are better identified, the nurse can develop more meaningful plans to meet these needs.

THE NURSING PROCESS

In keeping with the goal of this text—to provide the means for increasingly individualized patient care—attention is directed to the nursing process and its component parts: nursing history, nursing diagnosis, and nursing care plan (Fig. 4-1). The nursing process is a method of thinking, acting, and organizing whereby plans are based on individual patient's needs. An identified "need" requires assessment in order to develop the nursing action designed to bring about the care goal.

Nursing process is a systematic approach to nursing practice and

*Rothberg, J. S.: Why nursing diagnosis? Am. J. Nurs. 67(5):1041, May 1967. (Copyright The American Journal of Nursing Company.)

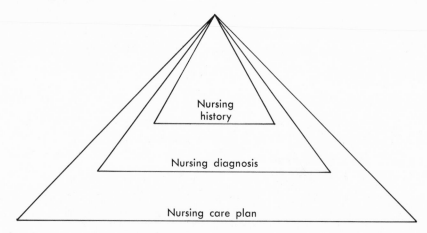

Fig. 4-1. The nursing process.

utilizes problem solving technics. Nurses have defined various steps to this process: assessment (interviewing, collecting data, and taking a nursing history); formulating nursing diagnoses, patient problems or needs; setting goals or patient outcomes; implementing nursing actions; and evaluating. In this chapter the terms "nursing history," "nursing diagnosis" and "nursing care plan" are used. The nursing care plan is a summary of the patient problems or needs and the action planned by the nurse. Evaluation takes place throughout the entire process and is an appraisal of the effectiveness of the care.

The nursing history

The first criterion for a nursing history is that it be in a structured written format. It is probably the most valuable written record in nursing. Such a document provides an individualized frame of reference for the guidance of nursing care throughout the patient's hospitalization. The ready availability of this information will enhance evaluation of any change in physical or behavioral response on the part of the patient, perhaps yielding clues to its origin. By using histories as basic reference material, nurses may be better able to predict changes in a patient's response or to anticipate similar changes in future patients.

Depending on the established procedures of the institution involved, the patient history interview is conducted by the unit nurse either alone or with the operating room nurse.

A history consists of specific data about the patient, data on which will be based the assessment of existing or potential nursing care needs. These data will also reveal the patient's problems relevant to the condition that brings him to the hospital as seen through the patient's own eyes. They may also reveal potential problems based upon a disparity between the patient's expectations and an objective, realistic prognosis.

A nursing history should include the following data: age, ethnic origin and cultural mores, socioeconomic background, religious background, medical diagnosis and proposed treatment, and the general physical and mental status of the patient. This is a minimal data list. More may be included depending on the facility and the type of patient care problems being met.

The history should be constructed to reveal the following items for assessment:

1. The amount of orientation needed by the patient in relation to the health care environment (Present nursing care will depend in great part on the patient's feelings and perceptions about nursing care experiences.)
2. The patient's feelings relevant to contact with family and friends during hospitalization
3. The patient's established habits of daily living (eating, sleeping, rest, elimination, personal hygiene), specific and immediate needs, and communication patterns (Subsequent care should be patterned around these usual needs whenever possible. Needs common to most patients are discussed in Chapter 2.)

Until expertise as an interviewer is developed, the nurse may wish to utilize the following suggested guidelines in obtaining the necessary information.

It is of singular importance that the patient feel encouraged to communicate openly and freely with the nurse. If possible, both the nurse and the patient should be seated in chairs. This eliminates the image of the nurse as authority figure, which is created when the nurse stands over the bedridden patient. It is imperative that the *nurse,* at least, sit down.

The nurse should approach the patient when there is sufficient time to be relaxed and available to the patient. The timing should also be such that the patient is not disturbed or distracted. Although it is of great benefit to involve the patient's family in care planning, the initial interview should be made without the influence of outside factors. The decision to involve the family will be based on the patient's communications regarding them.

Three questions will establish the orientation needs of the patient: Have you ever been in a hospital before? How long ago? Have you ever been in *this* hospital before? Once answers to these questions are obtained, orientation can be structured along lines necessary to meet the patient's needs. Orientation may need to be extensive or may not be necessary at all.

Questions to patients about nurses are generally answered in such a fashion as to bring visions of Florence Nightingale to mind! Most patients respond with comments about "how wonderful" and "how busy all the nurses are." Patient comments regarding the "busyness" of nurses and the nonverbal activities of the patient while making these comments lead us to believe that patients may fail to communicate with nurses in an effort not to "bother" them. Patients may also have suffered rebuffs by nurses who use their "busyness" as an excuse to avoid communication.

Many interviewers feel that freer dialogue takes place when the person being interviewed is not aware that what is said is written down. However, retention of data then becomes a problem. Therefore, the nurse-interviewer is encouraged to develop a "shorthand" system and to limit note-taking activities to a minimum while in the presence of the patient. These notes can be expanded at a later time. The nurse should also observe the patient's nonverbal activities and should note how the patient responds during the interview. Conclusions are then drawn from these nonverbal communications as much as from verbal ones. Asking the patient directly whether a nurse has ever done or said anything "bothersome" to him often illicits interesting, meaningful responses.

Discussion with the patient about his desired or expected contact with family and friends will give the nurse background information to use in the postoperative period. The nurse will then be able to incorporate the aid of the people most important to the patient in the care plans. It may be, however, that there are potentials of loneliness in a patient who is far from home and family. To another patient visitors would be a nuisance, in which case the nurse can make plans to assist him with this delicate problem.

It has already been stated that hospital routine should be modified whenever possible if it runs counter to a patient's established patterns and habits. Restatement of that belief perhaps will serve to impress the nurse with its importance in the overall picture for the patient. Individualized care would be nearly impossible to achieve in a rigid, inflexible, physical environment. However, when modifications are impossible in the best interests of the patient and the facility, an explanation will at least make the matter more reasonable to the patient.

The nurse now has a history. What does she do with it? The nurse will use the data from the history to identify patient problems and needs (nursing diagnosis) and to develop appropriate nursing actions. These actions must be planned around a specific care goal. Problems that do not require attention have been ruled out, and problems that require special attention have been brought into focus. A priority of nursing care problems has been determined, and the nursing actions to be taken have been identified. The nurse has had an invaluable opportunity to observe the patient's appearance and behavior, to assess his abilities and desire to care for himself, his vocabulary and language skills, and his learning needs relevant to his condition. The patient has also gained an orientation to his hospital environment.

The nursing diagnosis

The nursing diagnosis is an *evaluation,* as are all diagnoses, be they medical diagnoses prepared by the physician or the mechanical ones done by diagnostic machines. Specifically, however, this diagnosis is a *nurse's* evaluation of a patient's *nursing* needs. It is imperative that in making this evaluation the nurse base her evaluation of the patient on tangible,

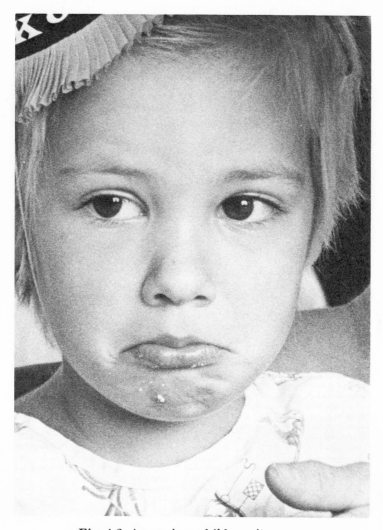

Fig. 4-2. An anxious child awaits surgery.

objective data collected in a scientific manner. Be it a frightened child (Fig. 4-2), a lonely geriatric patient (Fig. 4-3), or a person in obvious distress, the nurse's prime objective is to observe, analyze, and reach a decision. Thus, the nursing diagnosis is an evaluation based on current data (gathered during the nursing history interview) and covering certain physical and behavioral aspects of the patient's condition.

Why bother to make a nursing diagnosis? Nurses have functioned for years using the medical diagnosis as a base. Why not just continue on in this manner? Why not just go on carrying out the physician's orders and let it go at that?

The anwer to these questions is intrinsic in the goals of establishing a nursing diagnosis. These goals are (1) to identify the *individual* needs of

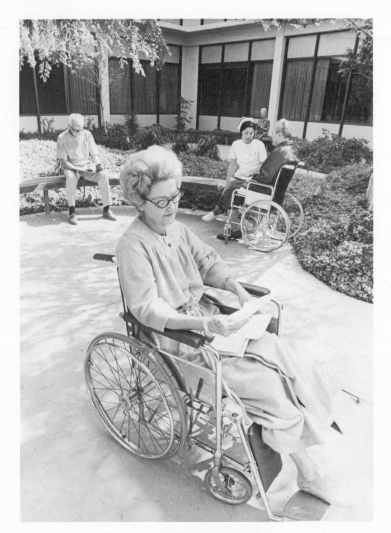

Fig. 4-3. Loneliness is an added burden to the presurgical patient.

each patient as a person and (2) to clearly define the *actions* necessary to meet these needs.

Another point becomes evident. Nurses believe that they deliver a unique commodity to patients. It has long been known that the hospitalized patient has needs over and above those provided for in the physician's orders. By making a nursing diagnosis in a formal manner, the nurse gives every patient the consideration due him in relation to the possibility that he may require special acts of nursing to aid him in his return to health.

Establishing a nursing diagnosis is mandatory to meet the premises on which this text are written. As previously stated in the Preface, effective nursing care requires that the patient be seen as an individual and not as a "case."

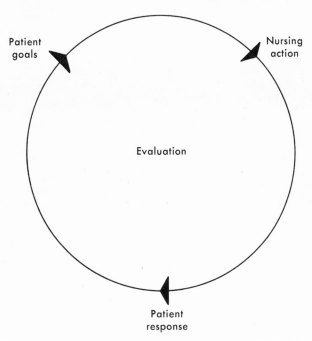

Fig. 4-4. Nursing care plan.

The nursing diagnosis will usually consist of one or two brief statements about the patient, reflecting his condition, behavioral responses, and needs. It is a concise summary on which nursing action is based. (Example: 80 y.o. ♂ for hip surgery; no family; high degree of anxiety; hx of COPD.)

A nursing diagnosis may also consist of a list of patient problems or needs that the operating room nurse considers relevant to the care of the patient in the operating room. Examples are: "stiffness of left arm from old injury," "hard of hearing," "is 5 ft. 3 in. and weighs 240 lbs.," "speaks only German," and "allergic to iodine."

The nursing care plan

In order for the nursing care plan to have meaning and function, it must be based on assessments and observations of the patient; present or potential nursing care problems must be recognized.[1] This is the reason that the nursing history, carefully taken and completely documented, must precede the formation of the care plan.

There are three points that every nursing care plan must minimally contain to have value: (1) patient goals, (2) nursing actions, and (3) patient response. As shown in Fig. 4-4, each of these components is related to the others. All are necessary for an effective nursing care plan; continuous evaluation of each must be an ongoing process.

Point 1: Patient goals. Based on the knowledge of the patient's medical problem and related personal facts, the nurse must decide precisely what she is trying to accomplish with the patient. Due consideration and attention must also be given to what the patient expects in the resolution of his problems. The ideal nursing goal of "returning the patient to a healthful state" must be realistically approached in terms of the presenting medical problem and in terms of the patient's potential for achieving an optimal state. Situations will arise wherein the medical condition will preclude a return to "normal" healthful functions. Therefore, nurses can be of more meaningful service if they will learn to identify and work toward levels *within the optimal goal* of returning the patient to a healthful state. The nurse must learn to identify immediate, reachable goals. For example, consider the following case history.

> Mr. X is a 70-year-old white male who is hospitalized for repair of an inguinal hernia. While obtaining the nursing history, the nurse became aware of two major factors that may pose potential nursing problems. Mr. X is a heavy cigarette smoker and has had two previous hospitalizations for pulmonary conditions. Mr. X also has no family in the area. His curt answers and general manner when discussing this lead the nurse to believe he is lonely and fears having no one to support him emotionally in the days ahead.

Achievable, realistic goals for this patient certainly exist within the concept of the optimal "return to a healthful state" objective. The nurse identifies the goal of preventing postoperative pulmonary complications and begins to plan time for teaching and practice of deep breathing and coughing exercises. The nurse discusses with the physician the need for pre- and postoperative positive pressure breathing therapy with recognition of the fact that this is an area of vital concern to the surgeon and within his province.

The nurse identifies another area of needed reassurance. She is able to find out from Mr. X that he has two good friends who appear to mean a great deal to him. He states that he would enjoy having them visit him in the hospital, but believes transportation would be a problem for them. The nurse determines in her planning that she will contact the hospital social worker to seek a solution to this problem. She also notes that she will contact the hospital auxiliary department and ask that plans be made for recreational activities for Mr. X.

This is one patient and one set of circumstances. Each patient will be different and have different needs; therefore, each set of goals and the steps necessary to meet them will be different. Examples of a nursing history and nursing care plan for Mr. X are found on pp. 45 and 46. This one patient is presented so that the process of looking beyond the obvious for obtainable goals may be better understood.

Point 2: Nursing action. The goals have been established and the present and potential care problems have been isolated. It follows that a workable care plan must contain a section defining the nursing actions that are anticipated to achieve these goals and treat the problems. Another asset in having the care plan in writing and as part of the patient's

NURSING HISTORY

Patient's name: Mr. X

Admitting date: 6/15

Date of history: 6/15

Medical diagnosis: Rt. Inguinal Hernia

History obtained by: J. Olson, R.N.

Nursing diagnosis:

70 yo. lonely ♂ in for elective abd. surgery; has pulmonary complications

General information:

1. Previous hospital experience: Yes _X_ No____
   Date of last hospital experience _1/70_
2. Previous experience in this hospital: Yes _X_ No___
   Date _1/70_ Service _Medical - Pneumonia_
3. Kinds of activities carried out by nurses that were helpful:
   "They were all just swell, but so busy!"
4. Kinds of activities carried out by nurses that bothered you:
   "Well, sometimes I felt I didn't move fast enough to suit 'em. I'm getting on in years, you know"
5. Visitor and family contact during hospitalization:
   Yes___ No_____
   (Desires for restrictions, listed).
   Doesn't expect visitors. Has no family. Two good friends - Mr. Roberts and Mr. Sanson, who have no transportation.
6. Patient's expectations of hospital experience:
   "To get my rupture fixed"

Established patterns of daily living:

1. Dietary habits: (include times of meals, snacks, dislikes and special preferences)
   7^{30} 12^{30} - 5^{30} light, soft diet due to dentures and constipation; states allergy to eggs, chocolate.
2. Sleep and rest habits: (include special needs for sleep)
   2 pillows - breathes easier; at least 2 blankets; usually retires at 12MN $\bar{p}$ TV news
3. Personal hygiene habits:
   Shower god taken in am; skin becomes dry if more frequent bathing
4. Elimination habits:
   Becomes constipated easily, uses Milk of Mag. ad lib, frequent urination, small amounts
5. Specific needs related to medical "complaint":
   Tx - preventative - for chronic chest, attention to diet and fluid intake re: elimination problems.

Questions asked by the patient:

"How soon can I go home?" (7-10d usually)
"Will I be put to sleep for the operation?"
(Have anesth. discuss $\bar{c}$ pt.)

Independent nursing observations of the patient:

70 YR. old Caucasian; wrinkled skin; appears "frail". Seems calm but became withdrawn from conversation (gazed out window); gave only "yes-no" answers when discussing family situation.
Has no religious affiliations.

NURSING CARE PLAN

Patient's name: *Mr. X*
Date of care plan: *6/15*
Medical diagnosis: *Rt. Inguinal hernia*
Surgical procedure: *Herniorrhaphy*
Plan made by: *J. Olson, R. N.*

Nursing diagnosis:
*70 y.o. lonely ♂ in for abd.
surgery; has pulmonary
complications*
Date of surgery:

Goals	Nursing actions	Patient's response
1. Prevent post-op pulmonary complications	1. Call Dr. re: IPPB; instruct pt. in coughing, deep breathing	1. Practiced 5 min. of DB-C p̄ instruction; co-operative; IT to be ordered by Dr. Smith
2. Provide emotional support through friends and hosp. auxiliary.	2. Contact social worker's office; contact auxiliary office.	2. Mr. X rec'd call from Mr. Sanson (friend) saying he would be in to visit him 6/17; Mr. X enthused et vocal about this visit

Routine treatments	Assigned to	Patient's response
6/15 1. IPPB x 5 min.	1. Inhalation therapy Dept.	1. Tolerated well, productive cough following Rx
2. Soft Diet	2. Nurse Aide Jones	2. Ate all of food on pm. tray
3. Surgical Prep Phisohex shower }	3. Prep. tech. to be checked by me	3. Small area of reddened skin p̄ shave; noted; will advise O.R.

Medications	Assigned to	Patient's response
1. Chloral Hydrate h.s. repeat x 1. ad. lib.	1. Self; adm. @ 10 "⁵⁄pm	1. 6/16—not necessary to repeat drug during noc

Suggested adjustments of goals and/or actions: (please date and initial)

1. p̄ operation will be necessary to splint wound during coughing; ↑ incidence rec. hernia in elderly pulmonary – complicated pts.   6/15   go.

ongoing hospital record is that it is then available to all of the nurses participating in the patient's care. Various people have various levels of expertise. The first nurse may be astute in identifying goals and the second nurse more astute in identifying actions to be taken. Little more can be added to the obvious fact that this type of planning enhances the original team approach already established as the premise of this text.

Point 3: Patient response to goals and actions. The final point that must be built into all nursing care plans is that which allows for, and will *encourage,* evaluation and readjustment of the plan. The nurse has established a series of goals and has directed the actions to be taken that will achieve these goals. Now the nurse must exercise skill in being objective and observant. How is the patient responding and reacting? Were the original goals valid? If not, they should be altered. If so, are the actions presently being employed actually achieving the goals? These questions must be asked frequently during the period of care and should at all times be uppermost in the nurse's considerations. Attention to this area will also provide an invaluable source of information for subsequent nursing research and evaluation of the quality of nursing practice in any given facility. Each individual can also benefit by periodic review of her own care plans and improve the quality of care by using these reviews as learning experiences. Quality assurance programs utilizing audit, peer review, and other processes are helpful to the nurse in assessing total patterns of care and her personal level of functioning.

UTILIZATION OF THE NURSING PROCESS
IN THE OPERATING ROOM

The ideal situation for the patient would be to have a surgical clinical nurse specialist available to each surgical patient. This nurse would function as the team leader, take the nursing history, make the nursing diagnosis, formulate the care plan, and allocate responsibility to various members of the nursing team. The clinical nurse specialist would also accompany the patient to surgery and participate in the operative procedure. This nurse would subsequently participate in the postoperative care and function instrumentally in helping to attain the goals established preoperatively. This is the optimal and ideal method of executing surgical patient care. It is highly individualized and personal, and it is specialist practice in every sense of the term. However, with present trends in health care delivery in which there is a marked increase in departmentalization of both medical and nursing practice, the ideal is not always possible to achieve. Until the physical restrictions imposed on nursing practice by shifts and technical duty loads are alleviated, it will be necessary to modify the ideal to better conform with the facility's structure. This must be done without sacrificing quality patient care.

In the approach to specialization, the operating room nurse functions

Name	OR NURSING CARE PLAN	
Age		
Scheduled operation	*(Sample pt. problems)*	
OR #		

Patient problems	Goals	OR nursing actions
Hard of hearing	Pt. will demonstrate understanding of instructions by: — responding appropriately (ex.—moving onto table) — nodding or shaking head — answering questions	Speak and articulate clearly and slowly; look at pt. when speaking to him or mask down; use of hearing aid preop if possible
Amputee (L) leg	Pt. will be maintained in proper body alignment in spite of amputation	Support stump in transfer to OR table and during procedure in slight hip flexion and internal rotation
Allergic to Morphine and Sulfa	Pt. will not be given any meds containing morphine or sulfa derivatives	Verbal communications of allergy to other team members Be sure label is on front of chart Be sure pt. is wearing special allergy identa band Check all drug labels before administration to pt.
Tremors of hands & shakiness in voice due to "uptightness"	Pt. will have steady hand grasp & calm even voice when talking, prior to induction	Be present and stay close to pt. Reduce noise, answer questions; use touch, body language & calm voice as reassurances
Ht. -5'2", Wt. -240#	Pt. will be transported & moved safely & comfortably; anesthesia time will be minimal; pt. will have no pressure areas or circulatory complications following surgery	Inform personnel going for pt. to have side rails of gurney padded & to have extra help available for moving pt. Elevate head for ease of breathing Have large instruments & retractors ready; plan for retention sutures Extra help in positioning & moving to table Have padded braces ready; pad pressure points well; examine potential pressure areas during procedure
Severe arthritis @ hip; unable to flex or abduct joint	Pt. will undergo D&C ē adequate positioning & exposure of surgical site, but ē trauma or irritation to @ hip	Prepare alternate position for D&C; confer ē Dr. Miles Have extra braces & supports available

Fig. 4-5. Patient problems, goals, and nursing actions, when combined with identifying patient data, become an OR nursing care plan.

as a participant and consultant on the surgical unit's care team. The unit nurse team leader will be responsible for the history and care plan. The operating room nurse will utilize the history and care plan in the pre-operative visit question sheet when the patient is interviewed. A sample questionnaire and the technic of utilizing it are discussed in detail in Chapter 6. The data in the operative interview parallel that in the nursing history and emphasize nursing actions peculiar to the sedated or anesthetized patient. The goals, as set forth in the care plan, can be noted and incorporated into the plan for patient care during the surgical procedure. This frame of reference again reinforces the team approach to surgical patient care; it is another method of reaching the goal of individualized nursing action.

The operating room nurse who truly plans for her patient's care will utilize information gathered by the unit nurses, but will want to go a step further and develop an outline of care specific for the patient while in the operating room. Fig. 4-5 is an additional example of a care plan format, outlining some representative patient problems, goals, and nursing actions. *Problems* are stated simply; *goals* or expected outcomes are written in observable, behavioral terms; and *nursing actions* are specific enough to be understood in the same way by any operating room nurse. This process follows the patient interview, assessment, and discussion of problems and actions with the patient.

Operating room nurses, in some hospitals, find it helpful to have the unit Kardex or meaningful care plan summary taped to the front of the chart. This provides some continuity and avoids the duplication of writing several care plans. Other operating room nurses use care plans with the two headings of "patient needs" and "nursing actions." The important point is that relevant information *be* passed from unit nurse to operating room nurse; of secondary importance is the particular card or piece of paper. Each institution can devise a care plan that is most helpful to its nurses and that results in the best nursing care for patients. The samples in this text are guides.

Again, it does not matter a great deal *who* does each of the items listed in the nursing process. It matters a great deal, however, that each part *is* done. As stated by Little and Carnevali:

> Care plans created from [the belief that each patient is different] do not eliminate the schedules of the first nurse, the interweaving of activities of the second, the routine orders governing the care given by the third or the understanding of the rationale of care by the student. Instead, there is the added factor of modification of care based on the unique response of each patient to the total experience of his illness.*

---

*Little, D. E., and Carnevali, D. L.: Nursing care planning, Philadelphia, 1969, J. B. Lippincott Co., p. 2. (Reprinted with permission.)

REFERENCE

1. Wagner, B. M.: Care plans—right, reasonable, and reachable, Am. J. Nurs. **69**:986-990, May 1969.

SUGGESTED READINGS

Coates, L.: Nursing by assessment, AORN J. **19**:1091-1104, May 1974.
Dodge, G. H.: Forces influence move toward nursing diagnosis, AORN J. **22**:157-158, Aug. 1975.
Fehlau, M. T.: Applying the nursing process to patient care in the operating room, Nurs. Clin. North Am. **10**(4):617-623, Dec. 1975.
Gebbie, K. M., and Lavin, M. A.: Classification of nursing diagnoses, St. Louis, 1975, The C. V. Mosby Co.
Kneedler, J.: Nursing process is continuing cycle, AORN J. **20**:245-248, Aug. 1974.
Kneedler, J.: Planning effective OR nursing care, AORN J. **19**:1243-1245, June 1974.
Little, D. E., and Carnevali, D. L.: Nursing care planning, ed. 2, Philadelphia, 1976, J. B. Lippincott Co.
Luttman, P. A.: OR/RR nursing record improves care, AORN J. **22**:909-912, Dec. 1975.
Marriner, A.: The nursing process, St. Louis, 1975, The C. V. Mosby Co.
Mauksch, I. G., and David, M. L.: Prescription for survival, Am. J. Nurs. **72**:2189-2193, Dec. 1972.
McPhetridge, L. M.: Nursing history: One means to personalize care, Am. J. Nurs. **68**:68-75, Jan. 1968.
Mehaffy, N.: Assessment and communication for continuity of care for the surgical patient, Nurs. Clin. North Am. **10**(4):625-633, Dec. 1975.

Roy, Sr., C.: The impact of nursing diagnosis, AORN J. 21:1023-1030, May 1975.

Rubel, Sr., M.: Coming to grips with the nursing process, Sup. Nurse 7:30-39, Feb. 1976.

Saxton, D. F., and Hyland, P. A.: Planning and implementing nursing intervention, St. Louis, 1975, The C. V. Mosby Co.

Smith, D. M.: A clinical nursing tool, Am. J. Nurs. 68:2384-2388, Nov. 1968.

Willingham, J.: Implementing individual patient care in the operating room, AORN J. 7:65-69, June 1968.

Yura, H., and Walsh, M. B.: The nursing process—Assessing, planning, implementing, evaluating, ed. 2, New York, 1973, Appleton-Century-Crofts.

CHAPTER 5

DEVELOPMENT OF THE SURGICAL CONSCIENCE

Surgical conscience is expressed in three major areas of operating room activity:

1. Interpersonal or psychosocial considerations: Identification of the nurse's role in achieving the best outcome for the patient having surgical therapy
2. Aseptic practices and technics: The principles of asepsis involving the environment with all its carriers of contamination, including the personnel; the choice of methods by which contamination is prevented
3. Safety of the patient: Planning for the patient's safety including his future safety; planning for the continued safeness of the operating room environment; protection of the staff and patient from electrical hazard, explosion, radiation, and exposure to other risks; ensuring the patient's safety concerning the administration of drugs and anesthetics

INTERPERSONAL OR PSYCHOSOCIAL CONSIDERATIONS

The basis of a theory of surgical conscience is *caring*. This means caring what becomes of the patient after his surgery is long past, caring how he views his hospital experience, and caring about his family. It is a kind of *vigilance*—a worry about possible hazards within the hospital. Examples of iatrogenic problems that the patient may needlessly be subjected to are noise[1], tracheal abrasion from an endotracheal tube, brachial nerve damage during anesthesia, and psychologic insults.

The results of psychologic insults may be totally invisible except for the withdrawn behavior of the patient. For example, sullen silence may be a sign that the patient has received blows to his ego defenses or that he mistrusts the ability of the medical establishment to help him. In spite of unbelievable advances in technology, the effectiveness of medical and nursing care still relies on the patient's belief in their power to help him.

A patient soon discerns any lack of professional interest in his problem and may respond by going into periods of depression which, though they may be justified, can actually impair his response to treatment.[2] The patient may become guarded and defensive in order to fend off the noxious stimuli that threaten his defensive patterns.[3] The nurse can give the patient assurance and strength and can make patients feel there is someone on their side in the struggle against pain, helplessness, and fear by helping them to verbalize their fears, listening to them, and responding to them with concern.

The noxious stimulus can be as small as a thoughtless comment about the patient's appearance or mannerisms made within his hearing[4] or as disastrous as giving the patient the wrong medication in the preoperative regimen. Such an error, if caught before surgery, makes it necessary to cancel the procedure and reschedule for a later time. A remark about another procedure can also cause the patient real distress. For example, a surgeon calls to the operating room nurse, "Better allow time for a radical dissection on that next one," as the patient is being wheeled by. Even if the remark does not refer to him, the patient may believe it does and will suffer accordingly as his imagination triggers assumptions about what will happen to him. This can happen by way of an "intercom" message from within the operating room to a clerical person at the central desk. The surgeon or nurse calling from the operating room may have no idea that the patient can hear and must be reminded of this.

The surgical conscience requires that any mistakes or failures be reported immediately on discovery in order to provide the patient an optimal chance for recovery and for therapy to benefit him in the degree expected. This takes not only skilled observation and reasoned judgment, but also *courage,* since at times the error is caused by unprofessional conduct on the part of other members of the surgical team.

Surgical conscience defined

A conscience refers to the *inner control* that directs its owner toward altruistic decisions. These decisions may take more time and energy to carry out than other alternatives, but they are based on the long range benefit to the patient rather than on the personal convenience of the members of the surgical team. A conscience presumes a system of *internalized values* and a sense of goodness and badness that prods its owner to work toward accomplishing the good and preventing the bad. Of all adaptive behaviors human beings have achieved, altruism may have the least survival value for the individual, but it is the very nucleus of a surgical conscience.

One of the most difficult paradoxes of human existence that the operating room nurse observes is that surgery and other treatments may provide for the survival of those least physically fit (in the Darwinian sense) and allow them a better chance to reproduce their heritable deficiencies than they would have had without medical or surgical intervention. However, a balanced view recognizes the importance to human existence of creative ideas and other human attributes not necessarily related to or dependent on physical fitness. The dramatic transplant procedures of the present, in conjunction with the future possibility of genetic manipulation, may offer every individual the best possible mental and physical well-being.[5]

The surgical conscience may tell us that we have not yet done all that we might do to be sure that the operative procedure is as well planned for the patient's present and future well-being as is possible. The nurse may even wonder if the best possible care is being provided. If there are doubts about any facet of the procedure, the nurse should be certain that everything has been done to make the procedure as safe, therapeutic, and expeditious as possible.

Our surgical conscience asks: "Is this the best set-up?" "Do I have everything that is logically necessary under the conditions existing?" "Will I need to be ready for unusual emergencies?" "What ought I expect in regard to this patient's surgery?" "If I were this patient, what would I want the nurse to do for me personally to help reduce the fears, nameless or known?"

The surgical conscience is often thought of as a rare blend of magical, unteachable qualities that include integrity, honesty, and outspokenness concerning any shortcomings in relation to the sterility of the field. It *is* teachable, however, and it is not magical. It simply recognizes that human beings possess a tendency for covering up their own errors, for ignoring risks, and for letting embarrassing faults go uncorrected.

Surgical conscience is behavior that consistently views the accomplishment of the patient's individualized surgical procedure as the product of the operating room nurse's work. If this procedure is to achieve all that it should in benefits to the patient, attention must be paid to maintaining excellence in psychosocial, behavioral, and immunologic details of the procedure, as well as in the physical details.

Application of the surgical conscience

Why would anyone conceal a break in aseptic technic? Perhaps one answer is related to the observation that the temperament of everyone providing care for the patient must be as controlled as possible. When things go wrong, revilement creates an atmosphere of hostile defense. Such a situation very quickly creates the added risk to the patient that the people involved will do anything, even use contaminated equipment, rather than risk further anger. If all team members could always be aware of the deleterious effects of rage and petulance, perhaps fewer breaks in technic would go uncorrected.

The ability to appear calm and to have a relaxed voice can influence every person involved in a crisis. Trust, openness, sincere concern for the patient, real respect for all co-workers, and a continual, meticulous surveillance of every detail of the work are important ways to bring about the proper working atmosphere in the operating room.

The patient is always the central figure throughout the operative procedure. The operating room procedural skills applied to the patient are the ultimate commodities the staff has to offer. Belittling the importance of technical skills has no place in the professional approach to operating room nursing. Technical skills are inextricably interwoven with interpersonal skills and with energy, speed, experience, judgment, and smoothness of motion. As a professional, the nurse uses her voice, facial expression, body stance and posture, individuality, and dexterity, to achieve order. For example, the nurse achieves order by calming the excited new staff nurse or quieting a frightened patient; there is order in the planning sequence of a complex procedure.

Uses of self. Operating room nursing involves continual therapeutic use of self[6] based on recognition of those behaviors that are effective in reassuring the frightened patient or the nervous operating room neophyte. Inept use of self occurs but can be recognized by its failure to elicit a positive response from the patient. The nurse who grins cheerfully at the patient on the operating room table just before anesthesia is begun and says, "You'll be just fine!" or "Don't worry about a thing!" may not be sensitive enough to see the negative patient response.

A study of cardiac patients indicated that comments having a basis in reality, such as "You'll wake up in the recovery room; your incision will give you a kind of burning sensation; you will have a bandage over your stomach," are useful in reducing patients' preoperative anxiety.[7]

Nursing research has provided indications that the postoperative course can be affected in several beneficial ways by thoughtful approaches to resolving some of the patient's worries and questions well before surgery. In addition, if the patient has a chance before surgery to practice those behaviors that will be expected of him after surgery, such as deep breathing, use of a positive pressure breathing machine, coughing, turning, crutch-walking, or limb exercises, he is better able to perform these postoperatively even when he is in a state of pain and distress.[8] Little if any learning can be accomplished in this regard if it is initiated for the first time postoperatively. The patient's energy can be guided to control his natural preoperative anxiety by allowing him to make active plans for his own recovery. During the preoperative day, the nurse may show him several ways in which he may help himself return to normal function after surgery.

Compromises in patient care. As previously stated, conscience is the sense of right or wrong within the individual. It is the awareness of the moral goodness or blameworthiness of one's own conduct, intentions, or character, together with a feeling of obligation to do or be that which is recognized as good. Conscience is instrumental in producing feelings of guilt or remorse for ill-doing. With practice, however, feelings of guilt for wrongdoing can become negligible. For this reason, the standards of performance in operating rooms and other patient care areas are not always the same. Some nurses are recognized as being conscientious and meticulous, and they consistently strive for excellence in all of their work. Others are satisfied with work that is mediocre or less.

How can the mediocre nurse be changed to demand more of herself? What or who defines excellent, mediocre, or poor work in the operating room? Little effort has been made to establish criteria in this regard. The actual evaluation is frequently based on the opinion of surgeons and their personal likes and dislikes, rather than on well-defined nursing criteria.

In reality, limitations may force the conscience to tolerate less than excellent workmanship. Such limitations occur when there are shortages of personnel, time or equipment, and materials.

Shortages of equipment. Equipment shortages may require certain adaptations to be made that will force the nurse to accept less than the perfect procedure that was planned. For example, a hip nailing procedure requiring a specially angled and unusually small sized prosthesis may be planned by the surgeon, who ordered the prosthesis well in advance of the operation. However, at the time of insertion it is found that a larger one is needed. In a large city it may be possible to send a messenger to borrow the correct prosthesis from another hospital. Frantic calls of this kind to other hospitals and to supply houses are not infrequent. In the small isolated hospital such a problem could be solved only by adapting the plates, screws, and prosthesis to the best possible functional position for weight-bearing and ambulation.

Special drills, saws, and dermatomes are difficult to maintain in perfect repair because their parts must be autoclaved for use at the sterile field. The ethylene oxide gas sterilizer, although not as destructive of equipment as the autoclave, leaves a glycocol residue after repeated sterilizations, which may be deposited in the moving parts and cause maintenance problems.

Conscientious attention to the maintenance of the thousands of instruments in every modern operating room suite is not a task for newcomers to operating room work. The nurse must appreciate the importance of meticulous care of eye and ear instruments and the need for making sure that cardiovascular clamps mesh perfectly. Instrument ratchets must be absolutely clean, and rust must not occur in the joints of instruments. Every instrument must be made and kept in perfect condition to do its proper task for the patient. A hemostat that pops open because of a defective ratchet allows unnecessary blood loss. If a vascular clamp holding the aorta during cardiovascular procedures were to open, the patient could expire, because the massive blood loss would obliterate the vessel and make it impossible to see in order to reclamp it.

Consideration of the meaningfulness of each detail in the process of

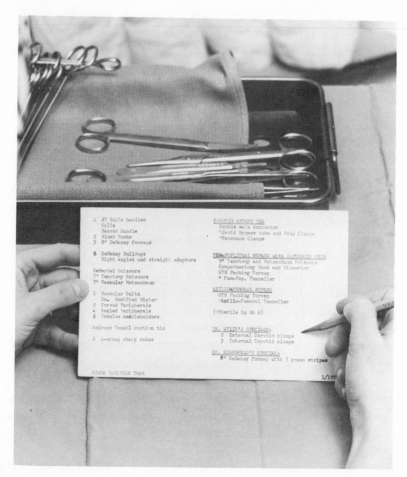

Fig. 5-1. Example of a standard procedure card used in surgery. Procedure cards are kept on file ready for use by all operating room personnel at any time.

operating room procedures should help the reader to understand that what may seem to be ritualistic tasks are performed by the operating room nurses with a deep understanding of their personal responsibility for patient welfare. Obviously the kind of preparation needed is ongoing, repetitious, and performed by teams. The fact that one nurse uses another's prepared set-up means that each has a clear idea of what is included in the selection of drapes, supplies, instruments, sutures, needles, sponges, and so on. Because time cannot be wasted in the operating room, since the longer the patient is anesthetized the more likely his recovery will be slowed, a standard list for surgeons' procedures is normally always available (Fig. 5-1). This standardization allows everyone to know exactly what is required. If some items are not available, this can be reported to the surgeon before the surgery, permitting time either to obtain adequate substitutes or to reschedule the procedure. Success or failure depends on efforts in preparation and readiness at all times for all types of procedures. In addition to surgeon's preference cards, it is possible to develop standardized *nursing* plan cards for specific procedures (for example, care common to all patients having vaginal hysterectomies, pacemaker insertions, and tonsillectomies). When both cards are used together, they provide guidelines for the operating room nurse in preparing the room and the patient for the surgical procedure.

Shortage of education. Shortages of education may have a more subtle, deleterious effect than shortages of supplies. An example is the operating room staff person who, through lack of knowledge, is not aware of the full range of possibilities in a given situation. It is usually just a matter of time for more learning to take place in the case of most normally motivated staff members. They soon become acquainted with the variety of alternatives as well as where and when each alternative is appropriate.

If, on the other hand, all procedures in an operating room suite are consistently performed in second-rate style and there is never any model of what constitutes first-rate operating room care, then, in all probability, none of the staff will reach full professional capability. Happily, however, the natural tendency for staff turnover militates against such a situation so that personnel are always exposed to fresh views and ideas. No operating room is left to its own methods without new personnel and new ideas for very long.

The supervisor, instructor, head nurses, and charge nurses must be the best obtainable. Teaching and leadership role models must be in evidence at all times on every shift so that high standards of performance can be observed by the learning staff, who in turn will make these nursing actions a part of their own repertoire.

Shortage of personnel and time. There are times when the surgical staff is overworked and exhausted because of limitations of personnel and time. Such conditions are always detrimental to patient care. The supervisor who frequently allows long hours without interruption, relief, or rest; late meal times; or other bad practices will compound any existing staff shortages by losing those staff members she has.

The operating room staff and the surgical conscience. The surgical conscience, at all levels in the hierarchy, recognizes and works to resolve those problems that lead to compromised patient care. It is a rare person who does not want to be accepted in the work situation and who does not want to do a commendable job if given the tools, the instruction, and the opportunity. Administrative and other controlling personnel who also wish to see the best possible care given patients in the operating room sometimes simply need to be informed of existing difficulties, methods that are outmoded, and the possibility of making improvements for the sake of patients in surgery. Well-reasoned suggestions for solutions to existing problems, even from the most recently hired staff person, should never be ignored. Rather, the suggestions should be taken as a barometer of staff enthusiasm for participation in the ongoing effort of the entire operating room team. Good leaders will receive many offers of advice and intelligent suggestions from staff members and in turn will act on them and reflect credit for new ideas directly back to the person who offered them. Useful ideas in the operating room gain acceptance because of their true value to improved patient care; they are not simply imposed upon the staff from administrative sources.

When rapport and mutual respect are established in the working staff of the operating room (and this is by no means always to be expected; it takes effort, interest, and *caring* to promote these attitudes), errors will be looked upon with compassion and support rather than with recrimination and the desire for punishment. The culprit suffers more from his own conscience than from caustic remarks of others. He needs no external punishment, because his sense of responsibility has already done its job and it is not likely that this error will happen again if he can prevent it. Internalization of such a conscience should occur in all persons who are responsible for the care of others, but especially so in the fast-moving, demanding, crisis-ridden setting of the operating room.

Although there are exceptions now and then to refute the following assumptions, it is nonetheless important to make a distinction between punitive, militaristic discipline and the gentler, more compassionate concern for the welfare of both the patient and the staff member. The staff member may suffer agonies of shame and embarrassment at his or her own blunders. Haste *does* make waste if one is tired and doesn't know what he is doing. Illness, fatigue, insecurity, and emotional upset among the staff can interfere with the best care patients ought to receive. When compromise is inevitable because of any of these reasons, it is still necessary to use a similar degree of judgment with the patient's welfare as the prime consideration in any decision. The problem of expedience under pressure of shortages of time, personnel, materials, or expertise requires as much study and preparation as any other recurring problem in the operating room. It is possible to plan for such exigencies and to avoid always being at their mercy.

Crisis philosophy. Rather than hope that the personnel, materials, and the time necessary will always be sufficient for the procedure, the surgical team can plan alternate ways by which the work can be done. The question might be asked, "What is the best way to resolve the shortage and still allow resolution of the problem?" Why leave such planning until the event actually happens? Part of the value to the nurse of experience in operating room nursing is the constant demand to utilize time, motion, energy, intellect, materials, and people to best advantage for the patient's welfare. Hairbreadth decisions are sometimes made, but the best ones are thought out well in advance of the emergency itself. The thoughtful operating room nurse constantly asks, "What would I do if . . . ?" An example: "What would I do if all personnel are scrubbed or circulating for surgeries in progress and an emergency cesarean section must be done at once?" In reality, one might use interns, medical students, nursing students, supervisors, or anesthesiologists—in fact anyone with any knowledge of the procedure to be done. In some cases the scrub nurse might even be taken away from an operation in progress if it is safely coming to a close. It would mean that this surgeon would have to find his own instruments and supplies (not an impossible task), which is not of much risk to his patient when compared to the risk of the obstetrical patient left to wait for a more opportune time. It is always a risk to interrupt the ongoing surgical team's concerted effort, even in minor surgery. However, instantly rating relative risk priorities becomes almost second nature to staff on evening and night shifts when operating rooms are notoriously short-staffed. This is a skill necessarily derived through experience and involves the integration of complex, rapidly shifting assessments depending on the unique situation.

The head nurse or supervisor of the operating room who is available by telephone at any hour of any day does much to reassure the working staff on duty; in fact, it helps to keep personnel from refusing these less desirable shifts. It is a mistake to assume that the staff on duty should disturb the supervisor only in the direst emergency situation. By then the staff may be too distraught to benefit from any advice the supervisor may offer from the relative calm of her home.

The "fire drill" crisis philosophy proposed here is part of the overall surgical conscience in planning for patient needs in most contingencies. It has been shown effective in military and public institutions, as well as in operating rooms of private hospitals. The philosophy is as follows:

1. *Identify all likely crises that have a legitimate chance of occurring in your operating room.* (Examples are cesarean sections; patients with ruptured aneurysms, gunshot wounds, head injuries, emergency tracheostomies, bronchoscopies; patients returned for control of hemorrhage after tonsillectomies, thyroidectomies, or heart surgery; cardiac fibrillation or arrest; foreign body removal from eyes or lungs; multi-casualty burn or blast injuries.) Include also the rarer emergencies, such as patients with poison bites of snakes or spiders, or bites of rabid animals.

Most important of all, and perhaps necessary to plan for in every detail, is the death of a patient in the operating room. Extensive protocol is followed, and the coroner's jurisdiction is also of concern. It has happened that the surgeon, in his consternation that a patient of his died in the operating room, demanded that the body be transported from the operating room back to the ward in order to avoid the coroner's visit! Often the coroner will not exercise his prerogative of coming in to examine the body, but his clearance must be obtained before the body is moved. Frank discussion and demonstration of how to prepare the body for the morgue are necessary for all staff members.

From the humanitarian standpoint, the next of kin, who may be waiting anxiously just outside of the operating room door, must not hear about the death of their loved one from anyone but the attending physician. Premature remarks from messengers or clerical personnel are out of place, even though they are intended to be sympathetic and supportive. The physician must assume this communication responsibility, although in rare instances he might assign this role to his assistant or to a nurse if other events prevent him from reporting to the family immediately. Eventually he must contact the family for an autopsy permit. Often this is done at the time the news is first broken to the family.

Personnel must know what to do about donated organs, proper disposal of dentures, prostheses, or other belongings of the patient. They must also know whom to notify, in what order, and how to reach them. All of these things should not only be clearly spelled out in a ready reference book but should also be rehearsed by the staff at intervals.

In crisis situations perceptions diminish, judgment fails, and reason may vanish altogether. When a fire is out of control, it is too late to start reading the directions on the fire extinguisher.

2. *Decide what emergencies require the quickest action on the part of the operating room staff; assign priorities on this basis.*

3. *Develop a detailed plan to care for each type of crisis* (without regard to the individual differences of surgeons); the plan should be flexible enough to use with any surgeon and any team.

4. *For each crisis that requires the most immediate operating room staff action, prepare a "crash cart" or tray* (Fig. 5-2 shows an emergency tracheostomy tray) containing all necessary items, sterile and ready for use. Preparation of crash carts must be accompanied by demonstrations and practice to provide the staff with the familiarity they need in order to locate, set up, and use the materials appropriately without a moment's hesitation. Use of the materials is explained and rehearsed in these demonstrations just as school children practice "fire drill" and Navy warships practice "general quarters."

Although the preceding discussion may appear to be an oversimplified, regimented set of suggestions, it was presented with a very definite purpose. This purpose is the ultimate reduction to routine procedure of all the possible crisis problems that may upset the equanimity or disrupt the clear thinking of the nurse in the operating room. Appropriately used, the suggestions and plans would provide the operating room nurse with a completely known response for most conceivable emergencies. This rehearsed response would be almost reflexly performed to the patient's benefit, *leaving the nurse in a sufficiently calm state to look after the more individualized needs of patients.* Nothing enervates the patient or upsets the operating room staff more than the sight and sound of a distraught, disorganized, or distracted nurse, trying unsuccessfully to provide proper patient care.

5. *Develop an "on call" list of nurses* who are willing to volunteer for

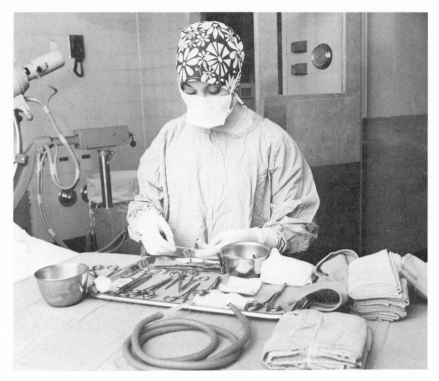

Fig. 5-2. Emergency tracheostomy tray is ready and sterile at all times so that no time is lost in assembling needed sterile instruments.

overtime. The quality of work performed by volunteers is usually better than that of disgruntled draftees. Many institutions have a rotating "on call" system whereby all staff members equally share this responsibility.

Value of the surgical conscience

The value of the surgical conscience is especially evident during crisis situations. New and untrained staff members can learn from the experienced operating room nurse who moves quickly, quietly, and with clear and economical effort. This nurse demonstrates to new staff the importance of organized, practiced, and skilled help in a patient crisis.

During calmer periods the inexperienced nurse can be helped to practice special routines that require dexterity and speed, such as the placement of Raney clips or silver clips on their respective forceps in neurosurgery, methods to keep from tangling the numerous sutures needed quickly in heart valve replacement procedures, or any rapidly moving procedure involving excessive numbers of tools and materials. In developing skills in crisis management the operating room nurse often becomes a very capable leader in many situations in or out of professional nursing.

In addition to crash cart regimes, the well-prepared operating room surgical care program provides "backup" systems and "fail-safe" devices so that there are alternatives for all vital equipment, personnel, and supplies. If, for example, a defibrillator is out for repair, another should be borrowed; personnel must have an opportunity to handle and become skilled in its operation, especially if it is different from the usual model. Standby equipment should be tested to be sure of operation in the actual setting. To illustrate the importance of this, consider the following episode:

> A special machine designed to store kidneys for transplant at a later date, perfusing them in transit, was brought to a small district hospital for the purpose of receiving donated human kidneys. No one thought to check the operating room outlets. At the last minute, when the machine was to be plugged into the wall outlet, it was discovered that the wall outlet was of a different type altogether than the plug on the machine. An emergency call was made to the night duty electrician, who solved the problem by taking the misfit plug off and attaching the wires directly to the power source.

Even though the problem was eventually solved, valuable minutes were lost and the recipient of the kidney may have had more complications than necessary because of the prolonged period of anoxia of the nonperfused kidney.

The difference between satisfactory and unsatisfactory work in the operating room may not always be obvious. But truly excellent professional work in the operating room relies on preplanning, meticulous attention to detail, tireless follow-up on staff education and motivation, and constant vigilance over maintenance of cleanliness and asepsis. More will be said about the latter concepts shortly.

The follow-up of nursing care plans devised by other nurses is another newer aspect of operating room nursing care. Charted and defined by colleagues, these plans may need clarification, implementation, or change, depending on circumstances and goals for the patient. As emphasized in Chapter 2, the patient must be viewed as a whole being—physiologically, humanistically, and behaviorally. This conceptual thinking is every bit as much a part of the operating room nurse's activities as it is of other nursing personnel who will follow the patient postoperatively through convalescence and possible home care.

In summary, the nurse might ask, "About what shall this surgical conscience be concerned?" "To what range of things shall we apply our conscience?" To answer, the ultimate goal is to afford the best hope of the fastest, least complicated recovery in all of its psychosocial and physiologic aspects for the patient. Such nursing care might not always seem to be the fastest or the most expedient, but the surgical conscience will not sacrifice accuracy, care, or feeling for the patient if they could negatively affect the surgical outcome.

Finally, a word about the conscience in relation to money and the saving of supplies. Although lately more conscious of the need to recycle materials, Americans have become waste-prone people, primarily because of

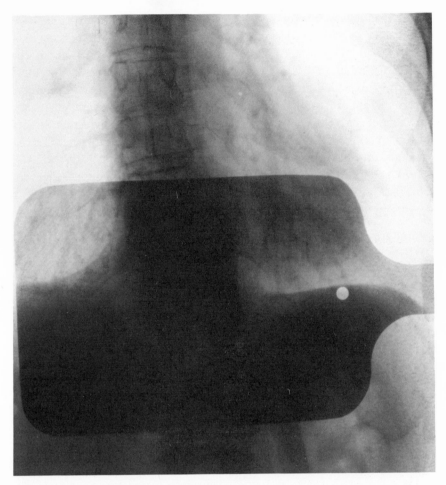

Fig. 5-3. X-ray film to detect gallstones is obscured by electrocautery ground plate. (Courtesy George Silva and Joan Tippett, Radiologic Technicians, Sequoia Hospital, Redwood City, California.)

expendables, disposables, and one-time-use supplies of all kinds. Such supplies became more prevalent when wages for human labor began to outstrip the cost of disposables. The patient's time, as well as personnel time, is now much more costly than these disposable supplies. Therefore, it is vital that caring for patients means saving the patient's money as well as that of the hospital. This is done by being accurate, efficient, avoiding duplication, or the need to repeat procedures already performed. For example, a roentgenogram to detect gallstones was taken while the patient was on the operating table; the film showed only the outline of the electrocautery ground plate, obscuring the area of bile duct and gallbladder that was to be examined (Fig. 5-3). Needless to say, the roentgenogram had to be repeated, using extra materials, time, and personnel, all of which added unnecessary cost to the procedure.

The surgical conscience, when implemented, often turns out to be simply *goal-directed behavior* and, in a sense, can be defined as the best possible surgical care of this patient, treating the patient as though he were a member of your own family. This goal-directed behavior involves thinking about what has led to the need for this patient's surgery, how he was prepared for it, and how he will be affected by it.

Concurrent thoughts of the operating room nurse must involve rehabilitation, as well as safety and repair. For instance, the dressing of wounds of the extremities in functional position is designed to promote rapid rehabilitation and uncomplicated return to normal function. This entails knowing the functional position for all extremities along with the means to achieve the position with the dressing materials at hand.[9]

ASEPTIC PRACTICES AND TECHNICS: STANDARDIZATION THROUGH RESEARCH AND KNOWLEDGE

Asepsis involves meticulous attention to housekeeping. It involves standard floor care and clean-up of horizontal surfaces and continual checking of sterilizing equipment to assure that it is doing the job it is meant to do. The endless details of folding, wrapping, and preparing supplies to be autoclaved are now commonly a responsibility of a central supply department; however, instruments and some supplies must still be prepared and sterilized in the operating room. Transfer forceps are no longer a necessary evil since almost every disposable comes in a presterilized pull-open wrap, ready for direct and immediate use on the sterile field.

All aseptic practices are designed to prevent contamination of the patient's surgical wound by bacteria. Even though it is believed that many of the postoperative infections are caused either by contamination of the wound by the patient's own skin flora or by previously existing infection of the patient, it is the duty of the operating room staff to apply every possible technic to prevent such postoperative infection. Skin preparation procedures in current use are varied, but most utilize some of the following chemicals in solution: nonionizing, detergent iodophors; halogenated compounds; phenols; quaternary ammonium compounds; and hexachlorophene. The use of an iodophor sudsing agent is recommended, working from the center of the proposed operative site (or area to be cleansed) outward. As detritus collects on each sterile sponge, it is discarded and another sterile one used. Scrubbing, the preparation of the hands and arms of those who will assist in the surgery, is carried out in much the same way working from nails to elbows with sterile brushes. Wraparound gowns with Velcro fasteners are an improvement over those with open backs to prevent contact with unsterile surfaces between members of the team.

The new laminar airflow systems being installed in many operating rooms are effective in filtering out a large portion of dust and bacteria in the air. These systems, first designed for spacecraft, use high efficiency particulate air (HEPA) filters to remove 99.9% of airborne particles 0.3 microns or larger. In conventional air conditioning air is exchanged 12 times per hour; in laminar flow it is exchanged 200 times per hour. Laminar flow is available in vertical or horizontal air flow. There are advantages and disadvantages to both systems.

With all the attention given to the maintenance of sterility of the supplies in relation to the surgical wound, the cleanliness of the environment, and the disposal of used items for careful decontamination before subsequent handling, it might appear that there will ordinarily be no postoperative infection whatsoever in the clean, well-run operating room. It is difficult to follow postoperative infections that appear 10 to 30 days (or even longer) after the patient has returned home. Yet stitch abscesses, bone infections, and other sequelae may be attributable to contamination at the time of surgery. Unfortunately, the reports of these incidents are sketchy and inconclusive, if not deliberately ignored to preserve the image of the infallibility of the hospital's aseptic practices.

There is continual improvement in packaging and design of all items for sterile application. The use of sterile disposables has obviated much of the need to boil, bake, or autoclave surgical supplies. However, none of these more primitive methods of reducing bacterial contamination can be

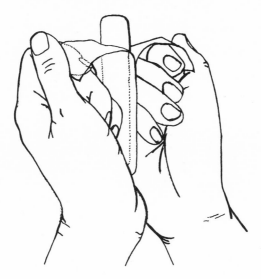

Fig. 5-4. Method of opening many types of commercially prepared sterile surgical supplies. The outer wrap, if unbroken, is impervious to dust and moisture and maintains the sterility of the inner pack. The opener's hands never touch the inner contents or the edge over which the sterile contents slide. By inverting the hands, the user can deliver the sterile item directly and quickly onto the sterile field.

entirely forgotten. Autoclaving (sterilization by steam under pressure) is still the most commonly used method of preparing sterile linens and instruments for use in surgery. Boiling in distilled water may be the method of choice for some implantable materials (Ivalon sponge) and for use when other methods are not available. The use of distilled water is necessary since ordinary tap water contains inorganic salts that react with tissues as foreign bodies and are therefore pyrogens (inflammation-producers). Strictly speaking, boiling water can only reach a temperature of 100°C (212°F) because water above this temperature evaporates as steam. This process is not sterilization, since it cannot kill all forms of spores.

Disposable packaging technics allow for handling and delivery to the sterile field so that ungloved hands will not come in contact with the sterile items inside the package. This is the basis of the "peel-open" package design for nearly all commercially sterilized and packaged items used in the operating room (Fig. 5-4).

Other wrapping technics should be standardized throughout the hospital so that all personnel handle and open supplies in the same manner. This requires practice so that the fingers do not slide over the edge of the container in such a way that the sterile item inside will slide over the contaminated edge. Beware the circulating nurse who opens supplies so quickly that neither she, nor anyone watching her, knows for certain whether she has touched the sterile item or the surface over which it traveled. Take care, watch, and be certain that you can see what you are doing in relation to all surfaces that should remain sterile.

Preparation of packs for the autoclave involves the use of freshly laundered cloth (double thickness muslin) of sailcloth-quality, strength, and weave. It is folded to provide tabs for opening without contaminating the contents. Many supplies and drapes are now commercially prepared in disposable paper packs of made-to-order specifications for one-time use. Some paper wrappers have an unfortunate tendency to "pop up" when opened because of stiffness of this material. Linen is more easily manipulated and will lie flat when unfolded but requires more expense to prepare because of laundering, textile lubricant, and examination for holes that would allow entrance of contaminants to the sterile interior. Hospitals maintain a wide variety of packages; plastic, cloth, glass, metal, and paper are the most common.

Principles of sterile packaging

To be safe for use in the operating room, any package design must adhere to the following principles:

1. *Allow visible evidence of integrity of the outer layer.* If glass, there should be no visible cracks or breaks; if paper, no visible tears or holes.

2. *Maintain a continuous integral outer sealed wrapper that will not allow entrance of dust particles.* It is well to remember that bacteria nei-

ther fly nor crawl, even though they are referred to as "bugs." Bacteria are *carried* on moving dust particles and on microscopic water droplets (such as those in aerosol sprays and in the material sprayed from oropharyngeal and nasal passages when a person coughs, sneezes, or talks excessively).

3. *Packaging materials should be impervious to dust and airborne microorganisms and resistant to wetting.* Commercial plastic outer wrappings are tested for perfect seal by immersion in a bacterial spore suspension and subsequent testing of the contents of the package for sterility. This is a very practical test of the integrity of such a protective wrapper.[10]

The basic principles of asepsis remain constant, but the methods of practicing these principles may vary with time, place, and philosophy. Sterilization is an integral part of surgical asepsis. The overall aims and standards of sterilization follow a general pattern:

1. The *production of sterility* by heat, chemicals, gases, radiation, or filtration

2. The *measurement of sterility* by using standardized resistant spores in random, periodic tests

3. The *maintenance of sterility* by dust-proofing, preventing moisture in or on sterile items, elimination of vermin, packaging, storing, and by the design of the package to allow extrusion of the sterile article inside without contamination

4. The *practical condition of sterility* by reliable sterilization methods; evidence that spores are consistently killed, proved by continued random batch testing; no demonstrable breaks in technic of the personnel performing the sterilization process; and, prescribed utilization, draping, gowning, and gloving technics

Fig. 5-5 contains all of the information necessary to fulfill these principles. Tested and based on many years of research by the American Sterilizer Company, these directions for sterilization are definitive for the routine care and maintenance of all materials normally used in the operating room.[11]

Principles of surgical asepsis

Surgical operations of all types are performed in the operating room because this location is kept virtually free of contaminating particles, organisms, radiation, and other hazards. If this were not the case, operations could be performed in any other location with equal safety for the patient. But in the United States, at least, hospital accreditation and accepted medical practice have set up strict building, safety, and practice codes that dictate the types of materials used to build the entire surgical suite, the size and proportion of the operating rooms, and the accepted practices to be implemented in order to maintain an aseptic environment at all times for the surgical treatment of patients.

PRESSURE STEAM STERILIZATION

How to prepare the load

1. Use freshly laundered fabrics. (This prevents superheating and provides longer life of the textiles.)
2. Limit the size and density of each pack. This ensures complete steam permeation and provides a liberal margin of safety (maximal size: 12″ × 12″ × 20″; maximal weight: 12 pounds).
3. Use double-thickness muslin (or equivalent) as wrapping material for surgical supplies. This provides protection after sterilization.

How to load the sterilizer

1. Place all packs (linen, gloves, etc.) on edge and arrange load in chamber so that only minimal resistance to passage of steam through the load will exist.
2. Place jars, canisters, and all other nonporous containers of dry material on sides, with covers ajar or removed. This permits prompt displacement of air and quick contact of steam with all surfaces of containers and contents. Drying is also facilitated.
3. Do not stack or nest utensils of the same size unless they are separated by layers of muslin.
4. Place utensils and treatment trays on edge so they will be sterilized and dried properly.
5. Place instrument sets in trays having mesh or perforated bottoms flat on shelves to keep contents in order.
6. In loads combining fabrics and hard goods, place the hard goods on lowest shelves of loading car. This prevents wetting of fabric packs from condensate dripping from hard goods surfaces.
7. Sterilize liquids separately from other supplies or materials.
8. Sterilize small items in baskets.
Note: Gloves processed in a gravity discharge type sterilizer should be placed in upper two thirds of chamber.

MINIMUM EXPOSURE PERIODS FOR STERILIZATION OF SUPPLIES, USING STEAM UNDER PRESSURE IN GRAVITY AIR REMOVAL-TYPE HOSPITAL STERILIZERS

	250-254° F. (121-123° C.) Minutes	270° F. (132° C.) Minutes
Brushes, in dispensers, in cans, or individually wrapped	30	15
Dressings, wrapped in paper or muslin	30	15
Dressings, in canisters (on sides)	30	15
Square-Pak flasked solutions		
75 ml	20	
250-500 ml	25	
1000 ml	30	
1500 ml	35	
2000 ml	40	
Glassware, empty, inverted	15	3
Instruments, metal only, any number (unwrapped)	15	3
Instruments, metal, combined with suture, tubing, or other porous materials (unwrapped)	20	10
Instruments, metal only, in covered and/or padded tray	20	10
Instruments, metal, combined with other materials, in covered and/or padded tray	30	15
Instruments, wrapped in double thickness muslin	30	15
Linen, packs (maximal size: 12″ × 12″ × 20″; maximal weight: 12 pounds)	30	
Needles, individually packaged in glass tubes or paper (lumen moist)	30	15
Needles, unwrapped (lumen moist)	15	3
Rubber gloves, wrapped in muslin or paper	20	
Rubber catheters, drains, tubing, etc. (lumen moist), unwrapped	20	10
Rubber catheters, drains, tubing, etc., individually packaged in muslin or paper (lumen moist)	30	15
Treatment trays, wrapped in muslin or paper	30	
Utensils, unwrapped	15	3
Utensils, wrapped in muslin or paper	20	10
Syringes, unassembled, individually packaged in muslin or paper	30	15
Syringes, unassembled, unwrapped	15	3
Sutures, silk, cotton, or nylon, wrapped in paper or muslin	30	15

How to take care of your pressure steam sterilizers

Daily: 1. Wash inside of sterilizer, using Calgonite solution. Never use strong abrasives, steel wool, etc. A long-handled cellulose sponge mop is helpful in cleaning the longer chambers. (Chambers should be cool before cleaning.)
2. Remove plug screen from bottom of chamber and free its openings from lint, sediment, etc.
3. Wash sterilizer loading car, using Calgonite solution.

Weekly: Remove plug screen and flush chamber drain line with hot solution of trisodium phosphate— 1 ounce (2 tablespoonfuls) to 1 quart of hot water. Follow with a flush rinse of 1 quart of tap water.

ETHYLENE OXIDE STERILIZATION OF MEDICAL AND SURGICAL SUPPLIES

Ethylene oxide mixtures are used to sterilize materials which, because of their sensitivity to moisture and/or heat, cannot be sterilized by steam under pressure or dry heat.

Warning: All materials should be quarantined in a well-ventilated area for a minimum of 24 hours following sterilization; however, aeration for as long as 7 days has been reported for special items. This is for the dissipation of the residual ethylene oxide gas absorbed by the material.

HOSPITAL EQUIPMENT AND MATERIALS STERILIZABLE BY ETHYLENE OXIDE

1. Telescopic instruments: bronchoscopes, cystoscopes, electrotomes, endoscopes, ophthalmoscopes, proctoscopes, etc.
2. Plastic goods: catheters, nebulizers, vials, syringes, gloves, infant incubators, heart-lung machines, etc.
3. Rubber goods: tubing, surgical gloves, catheters, etc. (Note: Pressure steam sterilization is the preferred method for these items.)
4. Instruments and equipment: cautery sets, eye knives, lamps, needles, scalpel blades, specula, etc.
5. Miscellaneous: dilators, electric cords, hair clippers, pumps, motors, books, toys, blankets, sheets, furniture, sutures, etc. Plastic film packaging material suitable for ethylene oxide sterilization: polyethylene of no more than 3 mil. thickness.

Fig. 5-5. Methods of sterilization. (From Sterilization aids, pamphlet prepared by the Education and Research Department of the American Sterilizer Company, Erie, Pennsylvania, 1968. Reproduced with permission.)

Safety codes include provision for electrical hazard and conductivity checks. Inspection for fire hazard, equipment and gas storage, and the clearance for emergency exits are but a few of the ongoing state code inspections routinely carried out in addition to the surveys of the American Hospital Association's Joint Commission for the Accreditation of Hospitals.

Observance of these basic legal responsibilities requires complete knowledge of how to carry out all of the practices defined in the codes. For example, sterilizer charts, which record the temperatures and pressures obtained for sterilizer loads over each 24 hour period, must be saved for 2 years. These charts are shown on demand to representatives of state public health authorities at any time they come to examine these records.

Complex systems are engineered to provide each operating room with particle-free air at positive pressure from a source near the ceiling to be

---

LOADING OF GAS STERILIZERS

Sterilizers equipped with shelves

1. All packaged items should be placed on the shelves in a neat and orderly manner.

Caution: Do not stack packaged items tightly. Always allow air space between packages.

2. Prepackaged rubber gloves may be placed in wire baskets for sterilization.

3. Avoid contact of load components with the walls of the sterilizing chamber.

4. At least 3 inches of air space should be provided between the chamber ceiling and the topmost packages of the load.

DO NOT REMOVE BOTTOM SHELF OF STERILIZER EXCEPT WHEN REQUIRED FOR CLEANING PURPOSES

Sterilizers equipped with loading carriages

Follow the procedures stated above. Exception: Packaged rubber gloves may be stacked in rows from back to front on the carriage shelves. Do not pack the rows tightly. Provide space between rows for circulation of the gaseous sterilizing agent.

CONDITIONS REQUIRED FOR STERILIZATION BY ETHYLENE OXIDE MIXTURE

12% Ethylene oxide	88% Freon-12
Concentration and exposure	650-750 mg/liter of chamber
	space for 1¾-4 hours
Total cycle time	2½ - 5½ hours
Temperature	125° - 135° F.
Relative humidity	40-80%

How to care for gas sterilizers

After each cycle: Determine functional efficiency of the sterilizer by examining the recording chart for deviations from data of previous cycles.

Daily: 1. Wipe chamber walls, shelves, and door with damp cloth.

2. Keep chamber drain line inlet (in combination steam-gas sterilizers) clean.

DRY HEAT STERILIZATION

Why should dry heat be used for sterilization?

Dry heat procedures are used when direct contact of saturated steam to all surfaces of the articles is impractical or unattainable. Materials and articles which should be sterilized by dry heat include anhydrous oils, powders, petroleum products, instruments which cannot be disassembled, sharp instruments which might be damaged by moist heat, and glassware. Since dry heat penetrates materials slowly and unevenly, long exposure periods are required, making it unsuitable for the sterilization of fabrics and rubber goods. Dry heat, in the form of hot air, should be applied in a specially designed sterilizer. Otherwise it is difficult to control within narrow limits.

EQUIPMENT

The equipment used for dry heat sterilization usually consists of a well-insulated oven, heated by electricity. Electrically heated ovens may distribute heat either by gravity convection or by mechanical convection (equipped with a blower for forced air circulation). The most efficient equipment for dry heat sterilization is the electrically heated, mechanical convection hot air oven.

LOADING OF DRY HEAT STERILIZERS

1. Never load the chamber to the limit.

2. Allow some space between packaged articles and between baskets or containers of supplies.

3. Keep all articles well away from chamber sidewalls, so that the hot air may circulate freely.

MINIMUM STANDARDS FOR DRY HEAT STERILIZATION

Although there are many varying requirements for dry heat sterilization, depending on the characteristics of individual items, the following standard exposure conditions are suggested:

> 340° F. for 1 hour
> 320° F. for 2 hours
> 250° F. for 6 hours or longer

Note: These temperature-time recommendations include a reasonable allowance for temperature lag in the load during the initial part of the exposure period.

CONTROL MEASURES FOR DETERMINING THE EFFICIENCY OF STERILIZING PROCESSES

The most dependable form of biological control is one which employs dry spores of a heat-resistant species, seeded in known populations on a known surface area and standardized so that a known survival time and kill time at a specific temperature can be demonstrated.

RECOMMENDED TYPES OF BIOLOGICAL CONTROLS

Pressure steam	Bacillus
(including prevacuum high temperature)	stearothermophilus
Dry heat	Bacillus subtilis (globigii)
Ethylene oxide	Bacillus subtilis (globigii)

FREQUENCY OF TESTING

It is recommended that bacteriological tests be conducted for every sterilizer in the hospital on a routine once-a-month basis and preferably at more frequent intervals.

AUXILIARY CONTROLS

Autoclave tape: Used for sealing the wrapper; indicates the package has been subjected to a certain degree of temperature in the chamber.

Chemical indicators: Inserted in the center of each pack; indicate that a certain degree of temperature was reached in that portion of the pack.

Note: All auxiliary controls indicate only that a certain degree of temperature was attained but do not indicate that the goods are sterile.

Fig. 5-5, cont'd. Methods of sterilization.

routed out of the room at floor-level exhaust vents. Without these systems dust and particulate matter on the horizontal surfaces would be continually borne by air currents rising upward from the floor. These particles would fall on the patient and the surgical personnel.

The concept of contamination. The concept of contamination was existent in pre-Christian times. The word "contaminate" is derived from the Latin word "contaminare," meaning "to bring into contact," "to soil," "stain," "pollute," or "corrupt," "taint," or "poison." It implies the transfer of a contaminating substance from one surface to another or to several other surfaces. Naturally, this concept preceded the germ theory of disease established by Semelweiss, Pasteur, and Lister, but the application of these ideas suited the later understanding of bacterial contamination by transfer of microscopic organisms through carelessness or ignorance. The housekeeping duties of early hospital nurses assumed crucial importance in the prevention of the spread of disease.

As time and technology have provided us with more thorough and efficient methods to maintain environmental asepsis, the individual nurse's role in maintaining asepsis has diminished in some areas but has assumed even more technical importance in the specialized area of the operating room. It is more efficient to have the sterilized surgical tools and the means and machinery to maintain an aseptic environment in one place than it is to provide these in many areas throughout the hospital. Therefore, all personnel in this one aseptic area are made familiar with the special needs and complicated technics required for the innumerable procedures now possible. Truly a specialization, operating room nursing has become a clinical technic of the most demanding type.

The concept of contamination involves contact between two or more surfaces, one of which has already been defined as contaminated. The surfaces may be composed of solids, liquids, gases, or any combination of these. For example, air currents (gas) may stir up bacteria-laden dust particles, which fall into sterile solutions (liquid) in open basins on the sterile table. The scrub nurse may touch the solution with gloved hand (solid) and transfer bacteria to the instruments to be used in the surgical procedure.

What kinds of things are contaminants? Any surface upon which *toxins, radioactive residues,* or *bacterial residues* are present. Such contaminants are removed by the methods best suited to the material as indicated in Fig. 5-5. According to the American Sterilizer Company in its "Sterilization Aids" (recommendations for effective use of sterilizing equipment), the factors associated with contamination and errors in sterilizer operation are:

1. Failure to observe and understand regulation of the sterilizer so as to maintain pressure of 15 to 18 pounds at sea level, equivalent to 250° to 254°F; and 27 to 30 pounds at sea level, equivalent to 270° to 275°F
2. Incorrect methods of packaging and wrapping of supplies, with no regard for size and density of packs
3. Carelessness in loading the sterilizer, with disregard for free circulation of steam
4. Failure to time correctly the proper period of exposure
5. Failure to carry out the correct sequence of operations in the sterilizing cycle; the result of carelessness, fatigue, or distraction
6. Lack of basic knowledge concerning principles of operation and care of the sterilizer
7. Tendency to shortcut because of pressures of work, distraction, or irresponsibility
8. Attempts to sterilize materials that are impervious to steam
9. Antagonistic attitude in place of voluntary cooperation on the part of the sterilizer operator

How is contamination of a sterile surface to be avoided? Contamination is avoided by isolating the sterile area, by maintaining possible contaminants at some distance away from the sterile area, and by removing or covering contaminated articles with sterile barriers. For example, in surgery of the intestine it is sometimes necessary to incise the bowel, which is considered contaminated all along its interior since it cannot be

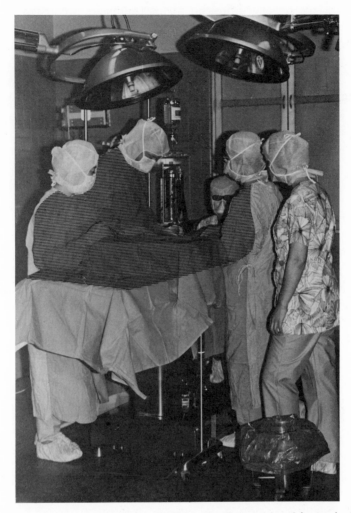

Fig. 5-6. Concept of the sterile field. The lined area in this typical operating room scene indicates surfaces and areas considered sterile. Other areas are considered unsterile. If any sterile surface comes in contact with an unsterile one, the surface so contaminated must be removed or exchanged for a sterile one.

treated to remove bacteria. When such an incision is made into the intestine, the knife, forceps, and other instruments used are immediately considered contaminated and are removed from the area as soon as possible. While the intestine is being manipulated, sterile towels are laid down all around the abdominal field so that bacteria will not be transferred into the open abdomen, but will be deposited instead on the sterile towels. Finally, when the intestine is again sutured, the contaminated towels are removed from the field and the surgeon and team members replace their contaminated gloves with fresh sterile ones.

How is sterility maintained? Many principles of motion, action, and sequence are observed in the operating room in order to preserve the sterility of the area near the operative site. Fig. 5-6 is a panoramic view of an operating room depicting sterile and nonsterile areas.

Basic principles of surgical asepsis are as follows:

1. *Personnel in the sterile area must remain in the sterile area* throughout the procedure. For example, sterile, scrubbed persons do not leave the room during the operation and, also, do not turn their back to the sterile field.

2. *Personnel who are not scrubbed must stay in areas at the periphery of the operating room,* a distance away from sterile areas.

3. *A margin of safety* (that small extra distance or space) is useful as a guide to movement and adherence to aseptic principles in each operating room.

4. Sterile fluids, equipment, or supplies are opened and delivered to the sterile surface without contacting the edges of the wrapper or container; *only sterile articles may touch sterile surfaces.* Edges of sterile wrappers or wrappers hanging below table level are always considered contaminated. *Tables are sterile only at and above table level.*

5. *Sterile fluids are poured carefully* so that they do not touch an unsterile lip of the container or splash droplets that strike an unsterile surface and then fall back onto the sterile surface. When pouring a sterile solution into a sterile container, the nurse should discard a few drops of the solution that have run over the lip of the container. This helps to ensure sterility of the solution poured into a container.

6. When reaching over a sterile surface, *an unsterile person must avoid bringing more than the sterile item over the sterile surface;* for example, the unsterile arm of the circulating nurse should not extend over the sterile surface when delivering sterile supplies. Remember, *when unsterile, do not lean or reach over a sterile field!*

7. Sterile drapes, towels, covers, and skin barriers are folded in such a way that *a generous cuff is provided for handling* by personnel in the sterile area. Persons wearing sterile gowns and gloves may handle these drapes and place them in position by grasping the inside of the cuffs. This protects the gloved hands and prevents inadvertent contact with unsterile surfaces that are being draped.

8. *Once placed in position, sterile drapes are never moved or shifted.* They are kept in place by towel clips or other fasteners; they are removed and replaced if contaminated by having been moved.

9. *Once gowned and gloved, the sterile members of the team may not lower their forearms below waist level.* Arms may be rested on dry sterile surfaces, but may not be folded with hands at axillae, for example. Moisture of perspiration may be carried by wicking effect from body surfaces up through the sterile cloth to contaminate the gloved hands. Technically, the sterile area of a scrubbed person consists of the front of the gown from shoulder level to waist and around the arms and hands. Unless it is

a special wrap-around gown, the back of the gown is never considered sterile. When passing each other, scrubbed persons always pass "front to front" or "back to back." A good phrase to remember is "sterile to sterile" and "unsterile to unsterile." In surgical asepsis, the words "dirty" or "contaminated" mean any contact with an unsterile surface, item, or person.

10. *A sterile person first covers the near side of any unsterile surface with sterile drapes, then covers the far side.* This avoids possible contact of the gown with the unsterile surface when a person attempts to reach across the area. When opening a small package on a large surface, for example, be sure the near edge of the wrapper covers the near edge of the table. An unsterile person opens sterile packages with the first fold away from herself to avoid contaminating the package contents.

11. *Talking is kept to a minimum in the surgical area* to reduce the spread of droplets. Even though the surgical team wears masks, excessive talking produces moisture droplets that are expelled with force in the process of articulating words. Many droplets escape the mask or are forced through it, especially if it becomes saturated with moisture. Masks should be changed at frequent intervals, between every surgical procedure, and *not* kept for use all day long.

12. *Movement and air currents around a sterile area are kept to a minimum to avoid contamination.* Personnel should avoid shaking linen. Doors to the operating room are kept closed.

13. All equipment, drapes, instruments, and sutures used in an operation are sterile. If an article becomes contaminated during the procedure, it is discarded. *If there is any doubt about the sterility of any item, it is considered contaminated.*

14. As outlined in Fig. 5-5, several factors determine the choice of *sterilization or disinfection method* to be used. These are:
   a. Type of microorganism to be destroyed
   b. Time in which to kill it
   c. Temperature to which the item can safely be raised without damage
   d. Cost
   e. Effectiveness
   f. Ease and speed with which it can be used
   g. Destructiveness of the method to item or materials

Nonobservance of aseptic practice as a function of human convenience

The skin is nature's remarkable barrier against all manner of inimical invaders. Besides protecting its wearer from bacterial, viral, or fungal invasion, the skin also protects against electrical current of fibrillating intensity under normal conditions of skin moisture.

When the skin is incised during surgery, direct contamination of the patient's bloodstream is possible. If all contaminating factors are controlled, the patient should not experience any prolonged postoperative febrile reaction. (Fever that persists after the sixth postoperative day indicates the presence of infection.) Routines for maintaining cleanliness of operating room surfaces with a germicidal detergent must be continually tested for effectiveness.

The design of the entire operating room suite should take into account the flow patterns of patients, personnel, machinery, supplies, and equipment. Besides control of lighting, air flow, and humidity, change areas must be placed in such a way as to control access to the operating room by anyone who has not first changed from street clothing and street shoes to operating room clean garb. This is a difficult problem for most hospitals. Operating room suites usually have a "back door" where personnel can go out in operating room clothing and come back the same way, bringing heavy contamination back with them from the hospital wards, the laboratory, or the cafeteria. The change area is a nuisance to surgeons who need to come and go frequently, as well as to orderlies who are sent hurriedly to the blood bank to rush back with the blood for the exsanguinating patient. In some cases, a foot-bath or mat dampened with disinfecting solution for wiping the shoes can prevent some cross-contamination. This chronic problem has yet to be resolved satisfactorily. A pass-through design in which the blood bank, laboratories, and x-ray department were very close to the surgical suite would be ideal.

If operating rooms and delivery rooms are combined, as is the growing trend, the problems of safety, communication, transportation, and exchange of materials and supplies are simplified. Costs are reduced, staffing is more versatile, and services are more centralized.

Human convenience must never interfere with safe aseptic practices. Consequences to patients and personnel must always be considered.

Routines in perspective

The processes chosen for prevention and decontamination of bacterial growth must be designed very specifically and in great detail to fit the need and the capability of the operating room suite. They then become *routines* in order to ensure accuracy, completion, speed, and total uniformity so that they may be done by anyone at any time, yet always in the same way. Table 1 is an outline of the basic aseptic routines.

Although the processes may become automatic in nature, personnel are cautioned not to become robot-like in performing these procedures. The good operating room nurse can perform the task but still remain receptive to new adaptations that will humanize the experience for the patient yet will not violate the principles of good technic. In devising routines for maintenance of asepsis, the goals are to achieve simplicity, clarity, definition, and reiteration of the activity based on known microbiologic principles. There is no place for casual thinking or performance when procedures are performed. They are indeed serious, but they need not be carried out without a sense of human consideration.

The surgical conscience, together with aseptic routines, is a formidable

Table 1. Aseptic routines

Prevention	Vector	Decontamination
Keep OR doors closed, reduce air turbulence Clean air filters, maintain positive air pressure into rooms Culture air samples in OR at regular intervals; if possible, review entire housekeeping routine for failures Use no powder in OR Use every means to reduce lint in environment; store linen far from OR	Air	Use of positive pressure unidirectional air flow control, HEPA (high efficiency particulate air) filters, changed frequently Careful clean-up of cast materials following use of plaster in OR Use wet vacuum pick-up technic several times a day to remove lint, detritus, hair, and other debris
Maintain rigidly controlled standards of floor and equipment cleansing with effective bactericidal, bacteriostatic solution (noninjurious to floor or equipment) Test concentration of bactericidal, bacteriostatic solution to maintain proper dilution Bacterial populations double every 20 minutes, therefore, preventive cleansing must be timed as effectively as possible to reduce this growth Develop a system for reporting and investigating postoperative wound infections Culture high-risk materials on a spot-check basis, e.g., anesthesia equipment	Particulate matter on horizontal surfaces	Meticulous cleansing of surfaces and crevices with bactericidal, bacteriostatic solution After every surgery, wash contaminated surfaces: OR table, arm boards, floor, suction bottles Use wet-vacuum pick-up technic: floor liberally doused with detergent germicide, then suctioned up by special wet pick-up vacuum machine Night time clean-up when rooms not in use: wash walls, floors, room furniture, lights; remember to apply silicone grease to OR table moving parts as much washing of the table tends to cause parts to stick unless properly greased
Personnel with infections not in OR Maintain minimum traffic of persons in and out of OR All personnel given thorough physical examination before employment in OR, and each year after Personnel never handle contaminated materials; wear protective gloves or use forceps Use gown, gloves, sterilization procedures effectively Keep skin, hair, nails clean and groomed at all times Keep shoes cleaned, wash laces (if any); replace when old and cracked Hair covered at all times in OR area; nose, mouth masked; no exposed hair such as sideburns, beard, or long curls; use of hoods recommended Masks changed frequently and between each surgical procedure	Personnel and patient	Remove and properly care for used gowns, caps, masks, shoe covers, equipment, instruments, anesthesia apparatus Cleanse skin surfaces, proper scrub technics for scrub personnel; careful skin prep for patient Circulating nurse washes hands frequently; scrub and circulating nurses always wash hands between procedures Report contaminating injuries (scalpel blade cut or needle puncture) immediately; obtain adequate treatment; remove blades and sharp objects for safe disposal Keep contaminated linen off floor. Dispose of all contaminated materials in such a way as to obviate any spread of contamination

Continued.

Table 1. Aseptic routines—cont'd

Prevention	Vector	Decontamination
Patient is showered with cleansing agent preoperatively; skin is given surgical prep before surgery with great care taken not to abrade the area when shaving		Maintain a well-understood, convenient decontamination procedure to be followed by all personnel after all surgery
Disposables preferred wherever high usage warrants the expenditure in preference to recycling processes, e.g., latex gloves, catheters, solutions, sutures, gowns, caps, shoe covers Store in undamaged wrappers in dry, dust- and vermin-free area	Disposables (Can they really be disposed of? What happens to the million plastic syringes used in a hospital year?)	Collect in safe, sealed container for ultimate burning or burying
Reusables preferred wherever low usage and high replacement cost warrant the reprocessing for repeated use Train personnel to prepare reusable materials accurately, especially glass syringes, and lumen of steel injection needles, stopcocks, manometers. Minute traces of debris autoclaved in these items may cause inflammation in tissue when used again	Reusables	Immediate terminal washing to prevent personnel infection or transfer of contaminants to clean surfaces

guard against infection, contamination, and their disastrous sequelae. Together they form the human protective barrier around the patient and, properly implemented, they are as effective as his skin in preventing infection.

SAFETY OF THE PATIENT
Mechanical and electrical safety

Environmental considerations. Common hazardous events in the operating room include inadvertent cuts on the nurse's or surgeon's hand by the knife blade, piercing of a finger by the suture needle, and cautery burns; uncommon hazards are surgical lights falling from their ceiling mounts, a surgical camera falling into an open wound, or the irrigation of the bladder with alcohol instead of water.

Unexpected and unpredictable hazards can be corrected only after they occur. Preventive care, however, can be planned and executed to avoid known hazards for both patients and personnel. For example, the objective of positioning the surgical patient is to allow most efficient access to the operative area for the surgeon. This positioning must be at an angle into which the surgical lights may be brought to bear from overhead and must allow the anesthesiologist access to the head and neck for maintenance of airway, for control of breathing, and for maintenance of a patent parenteral pathway. A safe position will also afford the patient adequate lung excursion, prevent excessive weight distribution on nerve plexi, and permit minimal pooling of blood with optimal blood return to the heart. A careful and thoughtful approach is necessary to meet all of these criteria of positioning. When this position has been achieved and before the patient is covered with sterile drapes, the nurse, surgeon, and anesthesiologist all have the responsibility for critically inspecting the patient from all sides in order to check all possible danger spots. In general each surgeon and anesthesiologist will have certain preferences.

Critical inspection means being doubly sure that the electrocautery ground plate is under a fleshy part and is not pressing on bony areas, particularly the sacrum. Many refractive decubiti begin from a combination of electrical, thermal, and pressure injuries in the area where the ground plate contacts a bony surface.

Moving, transporting, and repositioning the anesthetized patient involves knowledge that sudden shifts may cause severe hypotension. During surgery, blood volumes pool in the dependent regions and are slow to return to normal body distribution under the central depressant effect of general anesthesia.[12] Lifters and rollers that are designed to move patients smoothly should be utilized for anesthetized or recovering patients. The extremities must be examined to be sure that they are not pinched or caught in stretcher siderails or operating room table joints.

Broken needles, lost sponges, and other foreign bodies remaining in the surgical wound are the bane of every operating room nurse's existence. Rarely is the sponge actually left in the patient, but the event is so serious that it warrants the assumption that it *is* in the patient until it is found elsewhere. Foreign bodies left in the patient, even though sterile, cause severe pain, formation of adhesions, and, depending on location, interference with function. The standard radiopaque marker in all surgical sponges now makes it possible to locate the sponge by x-ray if it should be left in the patient. Unmarked sponges should not be used in the operating room.

Initial counts of instruments, sponges, needles, clips, or other easily lost items must be witnessed carefully by a second person. Wing nuts on retractors should be tightened firmly, and suction tips must be secure. The thoughtful scrub nurse develops many hand-eye-memory habits in order to remember where every item is at any moment during the operation. Routines are adapted to fit circumstances; for example, small sponges (4 by 4's) are discarded altogether in an emergency cesarean section or a ruptured aneurysm procedure, and only the largest and most easily retrieved sponges are used.

If a sponge is missing at the time of closure, immediate notification should be given the surgeon who may take time to search the wound carefully for the missing sponge before final closure. Re-entry after closure to retrieve a lost sponge costs the patient more surgery time as well as increased anesthesia time. Also, under these circumstances, the unhappy surgeon does not close as well the second time as he did the first.

Individual considerations. Safety involves the personal safety of the patients as well as preventive maintenance of equipment and environment. Electronic equipment, if properly used and cared for, can enhance the patient's safety. Electronic devices are not used as work-saving methods, but rather as a means of extending our perceptions of the patient's status. For example, electrical impedance spirometry for monitoring respiration during anesthesia, using specially designed equipment, offers a very clear assessment of lung function. One study shows that patients tend to lapse into respiratory depression when left alone in the recovery room; nursing attention and stimuli improve patients' tidal volume and ventilation.[13] As transistorization attains the ultimate level of miniaturization, the most sophisticated monitoring technics and telemetry may become commonplace in hospital care.

Vector cardiography may become sufficiently accepted to be used to detect the effects of mediastinal shifts on heart action or output when the anesthetized patient is turned or repositioned during surgery. This would warn the anesthesiologist of the need for changes in drug administration.

The use of electronic sensors, signal processors, and data control readout or printout systems is finding a place in health assessment. These systems provide more efficient routing of patients to the appropriate therapy without the need for professional medical services unless applicable.[14,15] In no sense can this be construed to mean replacement of the physician. There is an ever-increasing need for all qualified medical personnel, nurses, and health practitioners that is not likely to diminish in the near future. Skilled personnel are needed to extend the physician's reach toward effectively treating the patients who need him and to provide preventive health care services (such as inoculations, diet therapy, or follow-up home care) to those patients who do not need him. New approaches of all kinds, probably involving concepts that are unfamiliar today, will provide answers for the future.

The study of airflow, electrical apparatus, lighting, and acoustics will need to be added to nursing curricula of the future. There is already a trend to fill this knowledge gap with on-the-job training of the nurses in coronary care units, intensive care units, and nurseries for premature infants. These nurses are learning many sophisticated technics for the assessment of physiologic parameters. An urgent need exists to disseminate the appropriate degree of underlying electronic and biophysical principles so that nurses will have sufficient understanding of the safe operation and limitations of equipment in current use.[16] Guidelines for regulation of medical devices have been formulated by the Task Force on Standards and

Standardization of the Association for Advancement of Medical Instrumentation.[17]

How does the operating room nurse know when electrical equipment is unsafe? Certainly she does not wait until sparks are seen flying out of the wall outlet to call the electrician for repair. It is best to discover dead batteries in emergency battery-powered lights before the power fails! Power failure is another unpredictable event that can, nevertheless, be planned for in advance. Practice drills must be devised with the purpose of familiarizing staff with location, operation, and maintenance of the equipment. It is well to note the condition of the equipment at regular intervals and to provide for repairs, recharging, or replacement as needed.

Soon all electrical equipment installed in critical patient-care settings will be isolated from the vagaries of current delivered at the wall. This new approach to safety in electronic devices offers an almost ideal barrier to electrical hazards to the patient. Differences in ground potentials will not affect the patient protected by the isolating transformer. This device makes certain that the patient is grounded to one, and only one, ground, no matter how many electronic devices are applied to or implanted in him. The implanted or transvenous electrode from skin to heart has carried the most hazard, since these channels carry electrodes directly to heart muscle, which can be made to fibrillate with as small a current as 20 microamperes. Ordinarily, such a small current would do no harm outside of the body because the skin offers enough resistance to protect against small currents. The skin resistance fluctuates from 10 to 500 Megohms and its relative conductance and resistance are measured as the galvanic skin response.

Currents as small as 20 microamperes are sufficient to cause fibrillation of the heart when such a current is transmitted through the skin barrier by a catheter inserted directly into the heart during cardiac catheterization. A typical operating room ground-break detector is not designed to sense such minute currents. Integrated plans must be made to protect these patients in the coronary care or intensive care units, however. When such a patient is frequently transported hurriedly (for an emergency tracheostomy to be done in the operating room, for example), he is transported in his bed, which must be lowered and raised electrically. The wall outlet may be different ground potential than his pacemaker; the orderly leaning over to lift the patient may complete the circuit by touching the bedrails and the external connector areas of the patient's intracardiac catheters or the patient's EKG lead.

The patient with intracardiac catheters must be carefully protected, especially when emergency procedures require quick transportation to the operating room, since this adds to the existing hazard. In intensive care, coronary care, or other specialized areas, the multiplicity of electronic devices with skin electrodes or needle electrodes, which bypass the natural resistance of the skin, increases the chance that stray currents, even as small as 20 microamperes, delivered at the time the heart is in refractory phase (during diastole) will cause fibrillation of the heart. An ischemic heart is much more sensitive to trauma and will go into fibrillation in response to minimal irritation.

How does the nurse look for assurance that grounding is adequate in the operating room? In the past, the explosion hazard was of most concern. Now the greatest hazard is the much more sophisticated and subtle electrical hazard. The explosion hazard must not be underrated, however, for it is still present and is not yet a thing of the past.

Visible signs of existing electrical hazards are:

1. Cracks in insulation of wiring
2. No third prong (ground wire) in plug
3. "Cheaters" (adapter plugs) or extension cords in use
4. Electrocautery ground plates of inadequate size
5. Outmoded equipment of hazardous design (floor lamps, hot plates, electric heaters)
6. No regular electrical maintenance and teaching program throughout the hospital
7. Failure to employ a professional electronic consultant, part or full time, to advise the hospital staff on purchase, repair, and contract maintenance of electronic equipment and to provide for a continuing teaching program for the hospital staff on the proper use of all electronic equipment (If the hospital administration does not contemplate hiring a qualified electronic consultant, then it should also forbid the use of electronic monitoring or pacing devices for its patients. The technologic advances make it mandatory to provide both the electronic equipment and a skilled practitioner of electronics to advise hospital personnel in a wise and integrated selection of electronic equipment. This must be done without obeisance to any one manufacturer; the highest possible patient safety standards must be kept in mind.)
8. Disinterest and reluctance to initiate training and instruction programs in care and use of electronic equipment

Invisible signs of existing electrical hazards are:

1. Leakage currents caused by faulty construction or faulty design of the instruments. These can be detected with a voltmeter-ohmeter device designed to detect leakage currents. A program of periodic maintenance checks should be established for all electronic equipment.
2. Three-prong plug that has a break between the ground wire and the third prong inside the plug. Solution: purchase cords with transparent (clear plastic) plugs—now being manufactured for this very purpose.
3. Different ground potentials in different wall sockets in the same operating room. This can occur when repairs or remodeling is done and newer outlets are attached to different ground wire than the

old outlets. (The assumption that attaching a ground wire to a plumbing pipe will automatically ground the current is a fallacy. Newer conduit pipe is made of plastic [nonconductive] and is no longer a grounding vehicle. Worse, new installations underground may be made of plastic pipe while the ground wires attached to the above-ground metal pipe look as though they are ground-attached, but are not.)

4. The electrically operated hospital bed used by the incontinent patient with heart disease who is being monitored and paced. This is the patient for whom tne hospital budget should provide a built-in isolation transformer so that all current sources are derived through one output and grounded everywhere at the same potential.

What does the nurse need to know about electricity in order to make judgments about the existence of electrical hazards? What are watts, volts, amperes, and ohms? What do they mean in choosing one or another piece of electronic equipment to be used on hospital patients? Will the salesman from one company tell the complete truth about the shortcomings of his electronic equipment in relation to that made by another manufacturer? How can the nurse tell if the defibrillator is really delivering to the patient's heart the amperes that show on the dial? These and many other questions arise continually and should be answered by an electronic consultant for the hospital, not by a sales representative.

The ubiquitous "Bovie" machine, which uses the principle of high frequency radio wave desiccation, has caused more unnecessary tissue damage than any other single surgical instrument. Fortunately, newer concepts in design have now reduced the hazard of electrocautery. The so-called solid state instruments are much smaller and more efficient. The power output is isolated to protect the patient from electrical "overheating," the cause of burns at the site of the ground plate in the older nonisolated machine.

A less obvious hazard can occur because of antiquated plug and outlet systems that make it necessary for all modern equipment to be adapted by cheater or extension cords. In many instances hospitals of older design have been remodeled over the years and a variety of plug and outlet forms have been installed. As a result, a wide variety of cord attachments, adapters, and outlets is needed for ceiling lights, electric operating room tables, appliances, oscilloscopes, defibrillators, respirators, drills, and saws. Much confusion could be avoided if more attention were paid to electrical needs at the time contracting bids were accepted.

All outlets, plugs, and appliances should be standardized throughout the hospital so that any piece of equipment can be used in any other area of the hospital. This obviates the need for a panic search for the proper adapter. The large 220 volt outlets for x-ray machines are rarely in the places where they are most needed, so it is not uncommon to see a hazardous series of extension cords and adapters connected to portable x-ray machines in areas such as the operating room or recovery room. The outlets for x-ray equipment should be placed so that extension cords or adapters are not needed.

It cannot be repeated often enough that the operating room nurse can and must plan ahead, predict problems, and outguess and outwit those who would place patient safety secondary to budget, time, effort, or ego considerations. Compromises may be necessary in real settings, but priorities should always hold patient safety in first place.

Radiologic therapies and the responsibility of the operating room nurse

Although there are more than a thousand artificially produced radioisotopes, only about a dozen are currently employed in the diagnosis and therapy of human illness. The most widely used are cobalt 60, iodine 131, phosphorus 32, cesium 137, gold 198, indium 113m, and sodium 24.

What is an isotope? How is it made and why is it dangerous? How can it be both harmful and therapeutic at the same time? In contrast to other drugs, radioisotopes affect not only the patient to whom they are administered but also the attending personnel if the isotopes are not handled and controlled properly. Alpha, beta, and gamma (or x-ray) radiations are descriptive of three different types of particles, which have different trajectories and different penetrating power. Alpha particle loss, characteristic of uranium, is not as great a hazard to tissues as beta, and neither alpha nor beta is as dangerous as gamma radiation.

External radiation exposure of the body to penetrating gamma rays affects different cells, tissues, and organs in differing degrees. Blood-forming organs, gonads, and the lens of the eye are especially susceptible to radiation damage. As is true for bacterial and electrocution hazard, the best natural barrier against radiation is the human skin. Clothing, especially designed lead aprons, and movable lead shields can, of course, increase protection from radiation hazard (Fig. 5-7).

Alpha radiation of the skin without absorption through the skin is harmless, since it is completely spent at the level of the outer layer of cornified tissue. Beta radiation penetrates only a few millimeters into the upper tissue layers; very small amounts, if any, reach the underlying blood-forming centers. The outer layer of skin acts as a filter for the germinative layer beneath. Dosimetry, the calculation of range of radiation doses within which measured effects occur, is based on the amount of radiation known to reach the regenerative zone of underlying skin.

The objectives of protection from radiation injury are:

1. To limit exposure to external radiation to as little as possible
2. To minimize entry of radionuclides into the body by ingestion, inhalation, absorption, or through open wounds, when unconfined radioactive material is handled

Three factors determine radiation exposure from a given radiation source: (1) distance, (2) time, and (3) shielding.

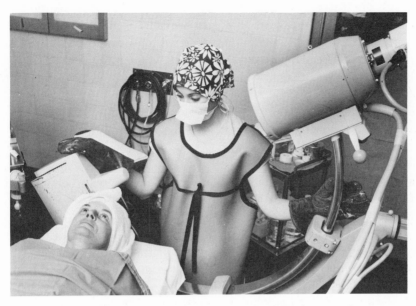

Fig. 5-7. Lead shield protection in radiologic procedures.

Protection against alpha rays is not necessary; protection from beta rays is adequately achieved by shielding; protection from gamma rays is achieved most effectively and cheaply by increasing the distance from the source. Radiation levels decrease as the square of the distance. For example, a person standing 10 feet away from a source is 100 times less exposed than he is when standing 1 foot away.

At this time there are three recognized units for three parameters of radiation effect: the absorbed dose (in rads), the exposure (in roentgens), and the activity (in curies). A curie is the quantity of radionuclide that gives 3.7×10^{10} disintegrations (or particle emissions) per second. This is the transformation rate of the substance and is now defined as its activity, not as a quantity. The special unit of absorbed dose is the rad, equal to 100 ergs per gram.

A roentgen (r) is a unit of amount of radiation. Defined in terms of its ionizing effect, 1 roentgen of radiation produces 2×10^9 (one electrostatic unit) each of positive and negative ions in 1 cc of dry air at standard temperature and pressure. It is useful only for x-rays of low or medium energy range. When higher energy transmissions are used, measurement in rads is more accurate.

Radiologic contamination. Since radioactive nuclides cannot be destroyed except by natural decay, decontamination of the air and water can be achieved by deposition, absorption, or adsorption. The material itself cannot be destroyed. If the material settles out in the bed of a stream or in the pipes of a hospital, the radioactivity is still present, even though the water flowing over it appears to be inactive. Liquid radioactive wastes are not discharged into the sanitary system indiscriminately but with due caution that the radiation level does not exceed the established upper limit. The slimes that are formed along sewage systems and the plants, fish, and birds that inhabit the sewage estuaries accumulate radioactive materials in their tissues at a far greater concentration than that found in the water itself. For this reason, federal and state criteria exist to monitor radiation contamination levels relating to the ecologic systems interrelating in the environment.

Concept of half-life. The term half-life is somewhat misleading. If the radioactive material is considered to have a life, why not speak in terms of its whole life? Why is this term used? The half-life is the time it takes one half of any given amount of radioactive material to decay. It is the time for the observed intensity to decrease to half of its original (first-observed) value, and it is characteristic of the nuclear species of elements. The particular nuclear substance, the variety of radiation, and the half-life are related to one another; knowing any two of these values allows calculation of the third. This is the basis, incidentally, for carbon dating of materials of unknown age.

Effects of ionizing radiation. Animal tissues such as bones and teeth, which contain elements of high atomic weight such as calcium, absorb much more energy from a given radiation than do soft tissues, which are composed mainly of elements of low atomic weight. All ionizing radiations have similar biologic effects, and these may be direct or indirect.

Direct effects. To produce an effect, there must be one or more hits by an ionized track on a sensitive target. The probability of effect depends on the probability of the requisite number of hits. There are far-reaching effects on the genetic code, which are then carried over to the daughter cells. Mechanically, these effects are stickiness, breakage, deformity, aberration, or fragmentation of the chromosome, with subsequent rejoining of the wrong pieces, and denaturation of protein within the chromosomes.

Indirect effects. The specialized structures of the cell, including the genes, are damaged not only by direct hits, but also by chemical products or by-products of radiation and ionization. Since the cell is 75% water and more energy is absorbed by the water molecule than by any other, the peroxides and free radicals that result from ionization of water are among the most important toxic agents involved in the ultimate inactivation of the cell structures. The loss of biologic control over cell division is the induction of cancer by radiologic means. This undesirable occurrence can appear in any tissue. Cancer of the skin was the first long-term effect of radiation to be observed. The length of time between exposure incident and the first appearance of cancer may be as long as 40 years.

Mammals are killed by exposure to less than 1,000 roentgens; fruit flies may survive 100,000 roentgens. Bacteria and viruses survive even higher doses, which provides the basis for the belief that extraterrestrial dust might contain disease-producing organisms. Cells injured by radiation may release proteolytic (protein-digesting) enzymes and nucleases (digesters of nucleus substance), which inflict more damage. The injury may be followed by scarring and inhibition of epithelial tissues with invasion by pathogens, inflammation, ulceration, loss of fluids, nausea, and diarrhea. Inhibition of blood formation leads to leukopenia and consequent susceptibility to infection. Anemia and its resultant defect in oxygen transport cause lassitude, anoxia, bleeding as a result of failure of platelet synthesis from megakaryocytes in bone marrow, and loss of immunologic capability.

Irradiation of a single organ can affect the function of other organs. For example, radiation of the spleen and liver retards synthesis of nucleic acid in the rest of the body. Irradiation of the pituitary can retard growth and affect sexual development and metabolism; it can also arrest proliferation of some hormone-dependent cancer cells, causing recession of such tumors wherever they occur in the body.

Sensitivity to radiation seems to be the greatest during the first 8 weeks of embryonic development. Exposure to radiation at this time may cause death or central nervous system aberrations not compatible with life: exposure to x-rays for diagnostic purposes during pregnancy may cause leukemia in these children in later years. It seems wise to say that the least amount of exposure possible to x-rays, gamma rays, or fluoroscopy is advisable. Growing children, who have more rapidly dividing cells, should avoid any kind of radiation if possible. These rapidly dividing cells, along with cancer cells, are more sensitive to detrimental effects of radiation. Pregnant women should be especially protected. As a rule of thumb, each rem received as a whole body radiation ages a person 2 to 15 days.[18,19]

Responsibility of the nurse. In the operating room it is especially helpful if the nurse understands what radiation procedures have been and will be performed on the patient coming for radiation therapy. There may be marks on the patient's skin in indelible ink. These are called "skin ports" and are used as guides to direct the beam of the radiation source correctly at the neoplasm within. The patient may feel stigmatized by these purple marks, especially since the prognosis for such patients may be marginal. When there is bone involvement, the nurse must use extreme caution in lifting or positioning the patient. The patient with a uterine or cervical radon implant can be forewarned of the expected postoperative symptoms so that she will not be overly upset when these occur. The systemic effects are those of radiation sickness with nausea, vomiting, anorexia, and profuse perspiration.

If radon seeds are accidentally expelled from the vagina of a patient, the thinking nurse remembers that radon has a half-life of 4 days, that it emits primarily alpha rays, and that shielding can be accomplished with a layer of paper. Naturally, the physician would be notified immediately since he may wish to take the patient back to surgery for replacement of the dislodged radon capsule.

The operating room nurse, as well as other staff members treating the patient, must remember to maintain interest in and hope for the patient.

The nurse must be aware of the regulations regarding safety in the presence of radioactive materials and the need for record-keeping to mark the time of insertion so that removal can be accomplished at the proper time. This knowledge will help the nurse feel at ease with the process of radiation therapy because there will not be uncertainty about these hazards. The nurse's assurance helps the patient cope with his fears about treatment outcomes.

Decontamination. If at any time radiation contamination is suspected or dangerous exposure to radiation is thought to have occurred, the radiation laboratory of the hospital should be called. In addition, a monitoring device such as a geiger counter or a scintillation counter should be brought to the suspected site in order to determine precisely what levels are present. Decontamination procedures can be started when the level, the type, and the exact location of contamination are known.

Leaching, repeated washing, and the use of soap and water are the immediate methods to reduce contamination. If these procedures are not effective, the use of titanium dioxide paste on skin surfaces is recommended. Care should be taken to avoid contaminating areas that were originally free of contamination by washing in such a way as to prevent run-off onto the clean areas. The eyes and the nasal and oral mucosa should be protected. When the decontamination process has been completed, a recheck with the scintillation counter should be made to confirm that the residual radiation has been reduced to safe levels.

The hospital's radiation laboratory professional staff has the responsibility of resolving all questions concerning the disposal of contaminated wastes, such as urine and stool. This professional staff also determines the proper disposal of linens, the length of time and the distance from the patient that visitors can be allowed, and the planning of operative care involving the use of radioactive materials.

The Atomic Energy Commission regulates storage, handling, transportation, use, and disposal of certified persons of all radioactive materials. The rigid controls are designed for the protection of the public and all who are involved in handling radioactive materials.

Drug and anesthesia safety

Safe use of drugs and anesthetic agents is an integral part of a surgical conscience. The ever-increasing volume of information about the actions and interactions of drugs and anesthetics makes it nearly impossible for a nurse to keep current in these fields. Various drugs and agents used in anesthesia are discussed in Chapter 7.

It may be helpful to the nurse to group drugs and anesthetic agents categorically and attempt to generalize the action of each category. This facilitates learning the most important characteristics of each group.

When administered, most drugs become reversibly bound to plasma proteins, presumed to be albumin. When another drug is administered that competes for the same protein-binding site, there may be a displacement of the first drug into plasma. It will then be metabolized by liver enzymatic action or excreted through the kidney or both. For example, apnea will be prolonged if succinylcholine is given with lidocaine or procaine. Succinylcholine is displaced from the protein-binding sites, and all binding sites are filled by the other drug. This results in excess amounts of succinylcholine in plasma, which leads to extended periods of depression of the central nervous system.

In general, anesthetics depress the activity of nerve cells and block transmission of the electrical impulse at the synapse by inhibiting the neuronal response to acetylcholine. General anesthetics depress the central nervous system regulatory mechanisms for respiration so that during anesthesia, if there is increased external airway resistance, the anesthetized patient cannot tolerate it. His tidal volume will drop without a change in the respiratory rate. Central integration and recruitment of respiratory neurons are inhibited so that they do not respond to chemical or reflex stimulation of the carotid and aortic body receptors or the medullary centers.

Anesthetics have a depressant effect on the myocardium. Renal blood flow and urine volume are reduced and sodium and water are retained because of the lowered cardiac output and lower perfusion pressure in the kidneys. Even though blood pressure is lowered by the general anesthetic, the blood flow to the skin increases by a factor of 2 during anesthesia; muscle blood flow is also increased. Body temperature usually falls. In older persons and in infants the temperature drop may be as much as 1.5°C or more. The depressing effect of anesthesia, the cutaneous vasodilatation, the use of muscle relaxants, and the transfusion of cold blood are a few factors contributing to this temperature drop. Severe heat loss during surgery may retard recovery. In adults shivering starts during emergence from anesthesia as the thermoregulatory function of hypothalamic centers returns. The act of shivering requires greater cardiac output and respiratory volume in order to supply more oxygen to the muscles; greater oxygen debt occurs with an increased acidotic state. Infants and older persons, especially, require additional, externally supplied oxygen.

Drugs may interact to cause effects that may endanger the patient. Ether and curare are synergistic; that is, each potentiates the effect of the other to cause a greater depressant effect than either by itself. All narcotics are potentiated by phenothiazine derivatives (thorazine, phenergan, compazine). Antagonistic drugs react against one another either detrimentally (as neostigmine versus curare), or beneficially (as nalorphine against narcotics).

Various barbiturates interfere with the anticoagulant effect of coumarin. Tranquilizing drugs used in psychotherapy may act with anesthetics to produce cardiac instability. Recent studies indicate that lidocaine and mepivacaine administered intravenously can cross the placental barrier. These drugs are taken up by the fetal circulation in concentrations of half that in maternal blood. Therefore, the pregnant patient and her unborn child may need to be treated with greater caution because many substances can and do cross the placental barrier to affect the fetus in still unknown ways.

Malignant hyperthermia, a rare but lethal phenomenon of anesthesia, is thought to be an atypical response to succinylcholine. If muscle rigidity instead of the expected relaxation is observed after the initial induction dose of succinylcholine, the response is considered very abnormal. Hyperthermia develops as a result of sustained muscle rigidity that must be counteracted immediately. The known mortality rate of this complication is 73%.

Two hazards associated with succinylcholine are bradycardia and asystole. Both cause potassium to flow out of cells and elevate the serum potassium level to nearly double its normal value. This can occur as quickly as 2 minutes after injection. This drug increases ocular pressure and is therefore seldom used in corneal or cataract surgery. The rising potassium level leads to cardiac arrhythmias, especially in burn patients or in patients with spinal cord injury.

Continuing inservice programs for operating room nurses in which anesthesiologists bring new information and review familiar concepts are of inestimable value to the patient; the informed nurse knows what to look for in order to protect the patient.

Waste anesthetic gas safety. Of great importance to operating room personnel safety are recent studies that have shown that inhalation of anesthetic gases in trace amounts over a long period of time produces birth defects or abortions in offspring of operating room personnel.[20] Personnel exposed to such long-term contact with anesthetic gases are alerted to this previously unrecognized hazard. "Scavenging" systems to vent waste anesthetic gases into the exhaust output of the ventilation ducts or into the outflow of the suction tubing are now available through commercial hospital suppliers. Operating room nurses who are pregnant should be assigned to other than scrub and circulating duties to reduce exposure to anesthetic gases unless the "scavenging" system can be shown to reduce waste anesthetic gases to less than 1 part per million for halothane and to 60 parts per million of nitrous oxide. Definitive regulations concerning venting of waste anesthetic gases are published by the National Institute of Occupational Safety and Health.

SUMMARY

An eminent San Francisco attorney, J. W. Ehrlich, in his book, *The Lost Art of Cross-Examination*,[21] makes a statement concerning legal responsibility in protecting clients that is applicable to operating room nurses in their professional concern for patients. He says that when you have another's responsibilities to meet, they must always be more important than your own. This conviction alone may serve as a criterion of measure to identify professional behavior in behalf of clients, be they plaintiffs or defendants in a court of law or patients in the operating room.

REFERENCES

1. Minckley, B.: A study of noise and its relationship to patient discomfort in the recovery room, Nurs. Res. 17:247-250, May-June 1968.
2. Sobell, D. E.: Personalization on the coronary care unit, Am. J. Nurs. 69:1439-1442, July 1969.
3. Wolf, S., and Goodell, H.: Stress and disease, ed. 2, Springfield, Ill., 1968, Charles C Thomas, Publisher, pp. 127-164.
4. Tao-Kim-Hai, A. M.: Orientals are stoic, The New Yorker Magazine, 1957; reprinted in Skipper, J. K., and Leonard, R. C.: Social interaction and patient care, Philadelphia, 1965, J. B. Lippincott Co., pp. 143-155.
5. Watson, James D.: Children from the laboratory, Prism 1:12-34, May 1973.
6. Ruesch, J.: Therapeutic communication, New York, 1961, W. W. Norton & Co., Inc.
7. Kennedy, J. A., and Bakst, H.: The influence of emotion on the outcome of cardiac surgery: A predictive study, Bull. N.Y. Acad. Med. 42:811-845, Oct. 1966.
8. Healy, K. M.: Does preoperative instruction make a difference? Am. J. Nurs. 68:62-67, Jan. 1968.
9. Artz, C. P., and Moncrief, J. A.: The treatment of burns, ed. 2, Philadelphia, 1969, W. B. Saunders Co., pp. 154-155.
10. Van Winkle, W., Jr., and Artandi, C.: Electron beam sterilization of surgical sutures, Nucleonics 17:86-90, Mar. 1959.
11. American Sterilizer Co.: Sterilization aids, Erie, Pa., 1968, AMSCO.
12. Minckley, B.: Physiologic hazards of position changes in the anesthetized patient, Am. J. Nurs. 69:2606-2611, Dec. 1969.
13. Noe, F. E., Bhatt, K., and Clark, H. W.: Electrical impedance spirometry for monitoring respiration during anesthesia, Anesth. Analg. 48:282-291, Mar.-April 1969.
14. Garfield, S. R.: The delivery of medical care, Sci. Am. 222:15-23, April 1970.
15. Chodoff, P., and Helrich, M.: Construction of an automated system for the collection and processing of preoperative data, Anesth. Analg. 48:870-876, Sept.-Oct. 1969.
16. Measurements and Data Corporation: Standards and practices, Electrical Safety 6(2): C-1–C-32, Mar.-April 1975.
17. Association for the Advancement of Medical Instrumentation: AAMI standards for electromedical apparatus, Diamond Bar, Calif., 1974, Quest Publishing Co.
18. Hollander, J.: Ionizing radiation and the cell, Scient. Am. 201:95-100, Sept. 1959.
19. U.S. Dept. of Commerce, National Bureau of Standards: Safe handling of radioactive materials, Handbook 92, Washington, D.C., March 9, 1964, U.S. Government Printing Office.
20. Cohen, E. N.: Cleaner air for the O.R.; Report to the American Society of Anesthesiologists, Washington, D.C., Oct. 1974. Reprinted in Modern Health, pp. 82-83, Nov. 1974.
21. Ehrlich, J. W.: The lost art of cross-examination, New York, 1970, G. P. Putnam's Sons.

SUGGESTED READINGS

Cahill, A. M.: Sterilization—It has a role in quality care, AORN J. 12:73-80, Oct. 1970.

Church, R. T.: Safety considerations for electrosurgical unit use, AORN J. 16:79-83, Sept. 1972.

Church, R., and Hamlin, W. T.: Electro-surgery demands OR vigilance, AORN J. 22: 903-908, Dec. 1975.

Committee on Infections Within Hospitals, American Hospital Association: Statement on microbiological sampling in the hospital, Hospitals 1:125-126, Jan. 1974.

Duff, R. S., and Hollingshead, A. B.: Sickness and society, New York, 1968, Harper & Row, Publishers.

Huth, M.: Principles of asepsis, AORN J. 24:790-796, Oct. 1976.

Litsky, B. Y.: Environmental control: The operating room, AORN J. 14:39-51, July 1971.

Litsky, B. Y.: Microbiology and postoperative infections, AORN J. 19:37-52, Jan. 1974.

MacClelland, D. C.: Laminar air unit: Achiever or appeaser? AORN J. 23:766-771, April 1976.

Mallison, G. F.: Housekeeping in operating suites, AORN J. 21:213-220, Feb. 1975.

Ngai, S. H., and others: Pharmacologic and physiologic aspects of anesthesiology, Anesthesiology 282:487-555, Feb. 1970.

Peers, J. G.: Cleanup techniques in the operating room, Arch. Surg. 107:596-599, Oct. 1973.

Ryan, P.: Basics of packaging, AORN J. 21:1091-1112, May 1975.

Ryan, P.: Inhospital packaging rationale, AORN J. 23:980-988, May 1976.

Sobel, D. E.: Human caring, Am. J. Nurs. 69:2612-2613, Dec. 1969.

Standards for: Draping and gowning materials; OR attire; OR sanitation; sponge needle and instrument procedures; preoperative skin preparation of patients; surgical hand scrubs; and inhospital packaging material, Denver, 1975, 1976, Association of Operating Room Nurses.

Thomas, E.: Bacterial hazards and control in anesthesia, AORN J. 19:88-95, Jan. 1974.

Thompson, R. E.: Static electricity—causes and controls, AORN J. 12:81-83, Oct. 1970.

Wisler, M. G.: Guidelines for use of ethylene oxide, AORN J. 19:1286-1295, June 1974.

CHAPTER 6

PREOPERATIVE NURSING CARE

Surgical intervention as a treatment for disease is rapidly becoming more complex. Future horizons are limitless in all fields of surgery as researchers move from the theory of surgery as a last resort to the transplanting of various organs such as the heart, lungs, kidneys, and liver. These organs now come from human donors, but in the future sophisticated mechanical devices may be used.

Patients in need of surgery often have several conditions for which they are being treated. Surgical intervention is not always the sole treatment for a condition, but it may be an important aspect of treatment.

The patient who agrees to be hospitalized has made a decision, either tentative or positive, to undergo surgery. He has accepted the physician's judgment that surgery is a necessary part of his treatment. Upon arrival at the hospital he will probably experience some misgivings and apprehension about the entire process. These feelings are part of everyone's inherent fear of the unknown.[1,2]

At a conscious level the patient realizes his need for surgery, and he responds to this by voluntarily entering the hospital. However, at the unconscious level the patient usually experiences fear, resulting in inner conflict and anxiety. This conflict produces the apprehension the patient feels as he is admitted to the hospital.[1]

Because the nurse remains in closer proximity to the patient than any other member of the health team, she can be particularly supportive to the patient by keeping him informed of the usual routine procedures he will undergo prior to surgery.

MAJOR CLASSIFICATIONS OF INDIVIDUALS RESPONSIBLE FOR PREPARING THE PATIENT FOR SURGERY

There are several major classifications of personnel involved in preparing the patient for surgery (Fig. 6-1). Under each of the classifications are many different types of people involved with the care of the patient. An example of this is the "physician" classification, which includes not

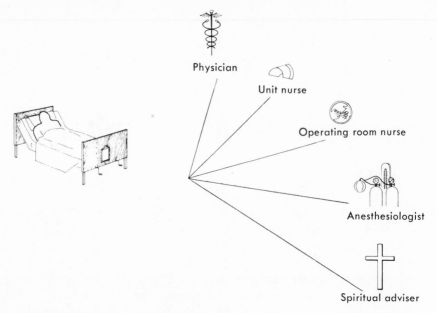

Fig 6-1. Team responsibility for preparation of patient for surgery.

only the patient's personal physician, but can also include the internist, cardiologist, radiologist, and pathologist. They can be either directly or indirectly involved with the patient's treatment. This chapter will consider these major classifications of personnel rather than each specific individual giving care to the patient.

The physician. The patient's first contact in the treatment of disease is the physician. In order to establish a diagnosis, the physician has conducted a battery of diagnostic tests. He will possibly explain the diagnosis to the patient and outline a course of treatment. Unless the illness requires emergency (immediate) surgery, most physicians will treat the patient using a medical or conservative approach. Should this treatment fail to cure or alleviate the symptoms, the possibility of surgery is considered.

It must be remembered that for certain diseases there can be no medical treatment; surgery is the only action and it must be undertaken immediately. An example of this type of emergency is a bowel obstruction or ruptured tubal pregnancy. This chapter will not consider those illnesses or diseases that require emergency surgery. These patients are usually in shock, possibly unconscious, and any treatment undertaken will be lifesaving. The patient is not as a rule in any condition to discuss his preparation prior to surgery.

This chapter will discuss the patient who is to have elective surgery as a form of treatment. Regardless of what the procedure may be—an appendectomy for chronic appendicitis, a radical procedure for a malignancy, or a heart transplant—each procedure is a major and serious operation in the mind of the patient.

The surgeon is responsible for informing the patient regarding his diagnosis and treatment, including all possible risks involved in the proposed treatment. He is also responsible for obtaining an informed consent from the patient prior to the performance of surgery. In addition to the consent that the surgeon usually obtains and retains in his files, the hospital requires a consent for surgery or other diagnostic or invasive procedures. This consent is generally obtained by the registered nurse after she has determined the patient's level of understanding regarding the proposed procedure. (See Chapter 3 for a more complete discussion of informed consent.)

The unit nurse. Upon admission to the hospital the patient's initial contact will be the nurse who will introduce herself and welcome him to the unit. She will then begin the formulation of a nursing care plan as discussed in Chapter 4. The nursing care plan is a vital link in introducing the patient to the nursing staff. The Association of Operating Room Nurses issued a statement identifying the goals of a surgical patient care plan:

1. To identify the physiological, psychological and sociological needs of *this* patient.
2. To assess these needs and develop a nursing care plan of action to meet them.
3. To implement a plan of nursing care which will provide a standard of excellence in the care of the patient before, during, and after surgical intervention.*

These goals are compatible with the care plan begun by the unit nurse and supplemented by the operating room care plan for those patients about to undergo a surgical procedure.

Although other health professionals contribute to the patient's welfare while he is hospitalized, none is so directly involved as the nurse who is the patient's first line of direct communication within the hospital, concerning his health problems and needs. This nurse must be prepared to meet the patient's needs during a time when he can no longer meet them himself.

The operating room nurse. The operating room nurse is unique in that she is the patient's advocate during surgery. Formerly her duties consisted primarily of "scrubbing," "circulating," or "assisting the surgeon." She was a skilled technician and usually a mechanical genius. The role of the operating room nurse has expanded from purely technical and mechanical functions to one that requires the ability to function in unusual situations by utilizing expert knowledge and professional judgment in assessing the problem and then implementing significant nursing action.

The operating room nurse provides services that contribute to the

---

*Association of Operating Room Nurses Statement Committee (Morgan, M., Atkinson, L. J., and Slavens, M. K., consultants): The first steps are crucial, AORN J. 12(1):43-44, July 1970. (Reprinted with permission.)

overall care of the patient before, during, and after surgery. The operating room nurse must above all be capable of exercising discriminatory judgment in the care of the patient during surgery when he is unconscious and unable to exercise control over himself. The nurse must be able to evaluate the patient's needs during surgery and then evolve and implement a plan of nursing action designed to meet those needs.[3,4]

The anesthesiologist. The physician anesthesiologist provides a supporting role to the surgeon. His function is to provide services that are vital to sustaining the life of the patient during surgery. He becomes involved in the patient's care plan when he makes a preoperative visit to evaluate the patient's condition as it pertains to the kind of anesthesia that can be most safely administered during surgery. The postoperative follow-up is conducted to evaluate the postanesthesia recovery. Any adverse reactions experienced during surgery are explained to the patient so that if any subsequent anesthesias are necessary he can report these experiences to the anesthesiologist.

The anesthesiologist will carefully study the physician's history and report on the physical examination of the patient. He will also question the patient concerning any previous anesthetics he may have had and how he reacted to them. Allergies are of the utmost importance, and the anesthesiologist will question the patient closely regarding any allergic or adverse reactions he may have experienced when taking medications and anesthetic agents or eating certain foods.

The anesthesiologist will perform a physical examination, concentrating on the circulatory and respiratory systems. He will chart his evaluation and grade the patient according to risk for anesthesia. During this visit he will carefully explain the routine that will be followed in accordance with his preoperative medication orders. The routine usually begins the night before surgery with the hypnotic and ends with the preoperative medications given prior to transporting the patient to the operating room. He will also explain to the patient the probable effects of the medications. An example of this would be the dry mouth experienced by the patient who has had atropine or scopolamine preoperatively. The anesthesiologist will allow the patient to express himself and to ask questions concerning the type of anesthesia to be administered.[5,6]

The spiritual advisor. Every patient should be given the opportunity to request a visit from his own pastor, priest, or rabbi. Those patients who have no particular religious affiliation should be informed of the hospital's own chaplain service. It is the nurse's responsibility to encourage those patients who exhibit unusual symptoms of fear or who talk morbidly of death to ask their spiritual advisor to visit with them. If they have none, the nurse can then suggest the services of the hospital chaplain. Every effort should be made to make the patient feel that there are those who care about him.

ROLE OF THE OPERATING ROOM NURSE IN PREPARATION
OF THE PATIENT FOR SURGERY

In response to the question of why the operating room nurse becomes involved in the preoperative preparation of the patient, Lambertson states:

> All practitioners of nursing must be capable of exercising discriminative judgment, explaining, executing and evaluating nursing care following the assessment of the needs of patients with potential or actual health problems. But the scope of these judgments is controlled by the knowledge, intellectual skills and abilities of the practitioner. Primarily, it is the difference in the ability of the practitioner to select generalizations and observations (theory, principles, ideas and methods) suitable to a particular problem or phenomenon and to use these generalizations and observations in the solution of the problem or analysis of the phenomenon.*

With the increasing complexity of surgical procedures and the advent of the surgical technician, operating room nurses will disappear from the scene if they do not begin to focus their theory oriented education toward the concept of total patient care. What does total patient care mean to the operating room nurse? The total care concept includes: (1) preparation for surgery, (2) care during surgery, and (3) postsurgical care. This spectrum of care can be used in identifying the role of the operating room nurse.

Nursing qualifications necessary for a successful
preoperative visit

The beliefs of nurses are summarized by deTornyay: "Nursing is an essential element of health care and nurses should be utilized to their fullest professional competency."†

Is the preoperative visit to the patient beyond the nurse's professional competency? Nurses today are being educated in theory, principles, concepts, and methods. Regardless of the clinical specialty chosen, the new graduate should be able to transfer the learned principles to any field of nursing endeavor. The patient has a "right" to this kind of nursing care.

Nurses need not be specially educated as psychiatric nurses in order to provide emotional support to the patient. They can usually draw on their own accumulated theories, whether learned in an academic setting or acquired from years of experience.[2]

The most important single asset necessary for making a successful visit is *empathy*. If the operating room nurse, while conducting the interview, is unable to put herself in the patient's place and understand his

---

*Lambertson, E. C.: Current nursing education and practice, Conference for Representatives of State Medical Societies Liaison Committee with Nursing, Chicago, American Medical Association, October 5-6, 1967, p. 7. (Reprinted with permission from the author and the American Medical Association.)

†deTornyay, R.: A "Flexner report" for professional nursing? Calif. Med. 113(3):81, Sept. 1970. (Reprinted with permission from the author and *California Medicine*, Official Journal of the California Medical Association.)

feelings, motives, and subsequent actions, then despite all her knowledge the nurse will be unable to provide the patient with any psychologic or physiologic support.

Another valuable asset of the nurse is the ability to analyze a situation and evaluate whether it is one with which she can cope or whether assistance is needed from other professionals. If in the course of an interview the patient presents a problem that the nurse feels she cannot handle, she should not be afraid to ask for assistance from someone more experienced. If the imagined problem turns out to be a false alarm, this should not be unduly upsetting. The novice operating room nurse will, as time goes by, accumulate her own experiences and theories. She will soon learn to recognize certain patterns of behavior exhibited by the preoperative and postoperative patient.[1,2] Some of these behavior patterns and nurse reactions are discussed in Chapter 9.

Assumptions concerning the patient

There are several basic assumptions to be considered concerning the presurgical patient. The first assumption is that the patient has made a decision to undergo surgery. He accepts the recommendation and judgment of his physician. Secondly, upon admission to the hospital he will feel some degree of apprehension, perhaps even a foreboding, which he may or may not accept as a perfectly natural fear of the unknown. It is the rare patient who can verbalize his ambivalent feeling about surgery, yet this ambivalence is operant. This is primarily because he has repressed his own natural antipathy toward losing control of a situation that involves his own body. Examples of this would be the loss of consciousness during anesthesia, the cutting of his body during surgery, or the lack of personal control over the events that occur prior to surgery.[1]

The third assumption is that the patient needs reassurance that everything will be done and everyone will be working toward his best interest. During the preoperative visit the nurse can do much to ease the patient's mind by carefully explaining the events that will occur before and on the day of surgery. If the surgery is extremely complex and will necessitate prolonged use of the postanesthesia room or will require that the patient spend several days in the intensive surgical unit, the patient should be made aware of this possibility.

The fourth assumption is that each individual is aware that he is alone. The support of his family and friends has been withdrawn; he worries about them, and he worries about his own aloneness. His outward concern often involves those he loves and he is anxious to alleviate their fears along with his own. The nurse can do much to include the family in at least a part of the interview with the patient, depending on the patient's desire to involve his family in this kind of interaction. The routines that are necessary pre- and postoperatively can be explained to the patient's family. Again, the nurse must be able to empathize or identify with the family, understand their fears, and help them adjust to the events that will occur during the patient's stay in the hospital.

Objectives of the preoperative visit

There are three objectives to any preoperative visit. The first is to reassure the patient concerning his operation. This is accomplished by supplying the patient with information about the various routines or phases of preoperative preparation that the patient will experience. The second objective is to instruct the patient on how he can help himself during the recovery phase. For example, patients who are to receive a general anesthetic should be taught certain prescribed exercises, some of which should be done as soon as the patient begins to respond in the postanesthesia unit. The third objective is that, through the interview, the nurse will be able to gather pertinent data that will aid the surgical team in providing a safe environment and relevant nursing care in the operating room, based on the knowledge of the patient as an individual.

In most instances all objectives can be fulfilled; in some cases, however, they may not be fully accomplished. Although there may be an occasional patient who will apparently defy the nurse's efforts at communication, the conscientious, interested nurse will use ingenuity to break through the barriers that may have been erected either consciously or unconsciously by the patient. The nurse must base her reassurance and teaching on the needs of the patient. He may want very little information or he may request a great deal. This assessment must take place early in the visit.

Principles of the preoperative interview

The preoperative interview must be tailored to each individual patient. The nurse cannot memorize a stereotyped speech and expect the patient to listen or learn anything of importance. The main point to remember is that there must be two-way communication. The nurse talks for a while and then listens while the patient talks. Listening is an art that can be cultivated by any nurse who wishes to be a skillful interviewer. If, instead of listening, the nurse is planning the next speech, the patient's unspoken plea for help will never be heard. Most of the anxieties and fears a patient feels are not transmitted by words, but by nonverbal means. The nurse listens with her eyes as well as with her ears.

Preoperative visits can be conducted using a variety of methods. Hospitals with light operating room schedules may have all surgical patients interviewed; others with heavy schedules may select for interviewing only those patients who will undergo "major" surgical procedures; some hospitals have group preoperative classes. The method for choosing patients to be interviewed should be made a written procedure and should be utilized in the orientation of all registered nurses.

This orientation should be designed to fit the circumstances in each institutional setting. There are a variety of methods used in orienting personnel in patient interviewing. One such method is seen in commercially available audiovisual aids dealing with patient interviewing, which can be adapted to fit various situations.

Another effective method is role playing with staff members selected to be "patients." In this method the group provides feedback after each "patient" interview. Auxiliary staff provide many challenges to nurses when they are asked to participate in the role of "patient." Each "patient" is given a card with his name, age, diagnosis, marital status, and enough personal data to make him real. The nurse receives only the information that would ordinarily be found in the surgery schedule. The members of the group critique the performance on the basis of how they would have responded in a similar situation. Role playing allows nurses to develop their own approach and to refine it by practice with their colleagues.

Patient interviews usually take place on the day prior to surgery. If the patient has been an "in-patient" for several days, there will usually be no problem arranging time for the preoperative visit. It becomes increasingly more difficult to arrange time for a satisfactory visit when the patient is admitted late in the afternoon on the day before surgery. Some people become physically tired and emotionally frustrated by the admitting process itself. When they are also anticipating surgery the following day, the increased tension may cause them to react negatively to the preoperative interview. The nurse should be aware of the various interactions that can occur in such situations and be prepared to cope with them. Several references found at the end of the chapter will aid in planning a course of action.

A vital point to remember is that the interview or group class is not just an information giving and gathering session; it is also a means of establishing rapport and providing support to the patient and his family.

The interview

Before beginning the daily preoperative visits, the nurse checks the surgery schedule and makes a list of the names of the patients she plans to include in her visits. A tool that can be used to expedite the visit, by helping to structure the interview, is begun in the operating room by the nurse or ward clerk. Some nurses design their own interview guidelines after they have set up interviewing protocols. When the "patient identification data" portion of the sheet has been completed, the nurse starts the visit with a review of the patient's chart and a discussion of the care plan with the unit nurse (Fig. 6-2).

Chart data are then transferred to the interview sheet, and the nurse is ready to meet the patient.

Entering the patient's room, the nurse greets the patient by name and introduces herself. She explains the purpose of her visit and inquires whether the time is convenient for an interview. When visitors are pres-

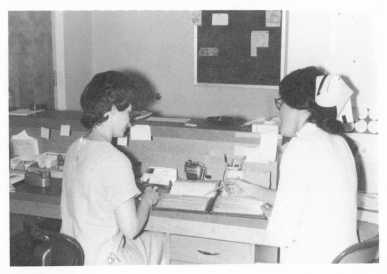

Fig. 6-2. Operating room nurse and unit head nurse review the nursing care plan.

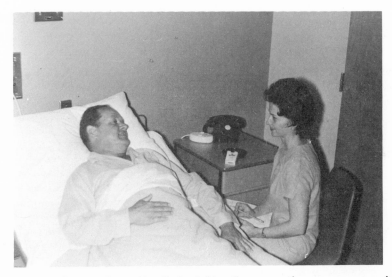

Fig. 6-3. By sitting at the patient's bedside, the operating room nurse indicates that the patient has her undivided attention.

ent, the nurse should let the patient know that he can ask the nurse to return later or that he can include his visitors in the interview. The patient will more frequently tend to include visitors, especially if they are members of the immediate family.

The patient's initial response should reveal his knowledge of the scheduled surgery and his willingness to be interviewed. Before starting, the nurse draws up a chair and sits down (Fig. 6-3). This indicates to the

OPERATING ROOM NURSES INTERVIEW SHEET

Patient's name _Ray Wilkins_   Date _9/6_   Interviewer _M Jones_

Hosp. no. _776-5942_   Room no. _640_   Age _50_   Sex _Male_

Operation _Cholecystectomy_   Date of surgery _9/7_   Time _0900_

Surgeon _Wright_   Attending Dr. _Smith_   Anesthesiologist _Samson_

Areas of patient need	Action taken by OR nurse
1. History: Allergies: _Penicillin - tape - some foods_ Dentures: _Full mouth - refuses to take out_ Prosthesis: _Denies hair piece - contact lens_ Previous surgery: _Lumbar laminectomy and fusion 1970_ Major accidents: _None_ Physical problems: _C/o low back pain and lack of flexibility of the spine_	_Check for possible hair piece and hearing aid._ _Remind Dr. Samson about the dentures - also that the patient is one of Jehovah's witnesses and has signed refusal to take blood form._ _Place small pillow under his knees or flex table to relieve tension on his back._ _Use paper tape._
2. Safety observations: Language: _English_ Audio: _poor c̄ hearing aid_ Comprehension: _good if not too technical_	_Pt very hard of hearing - be sure to have his attention when explaining procedures_ _Do not use technical terms_ _Explain what you are doing if he's not sedated._
3. Social: Spouse: _Ethel - married 30 yrs_ Children: _John - 29 - lives Arizona - Pat. 25 lives in town - one child_ Problems: _wife is semi invalid. Pt very concerned that daughter will not check on her (Social worker to see what can be done)_	_His wife and daughter will be waiting in the family room for Dr. Wright & Smith_
4. Other: Emotional status: _expresses some anxiety - probably less than he feels - needs reassurance_ Spiritual status: _Jehovah's witnesses - accepts all medical aid but refuses blood transfusions_ Special procedures: _Insertion of Levine tube before surgery_ Drains/catheters: _Penrose drain - explained._	_Although he expresses concern and is somewhat fearful, he is very firm in his faith and fully understands the risks involved by refusal of blood transfusions if needed. If explanations are given, will be very cooperative._

5. Instructions preop: Explain sequence of events which are routine for preop patients. Use terminology familiar to the patient. Refer specialized questions to the proper source. Instructions postop: Explain, demonstrate, and have patient give a return demonstration of appropriate postop exercises, i.e., deep breathing, turning, leg and foot exercises, and the proper method of getting out of bed. Each exercise dependent on the type of surgery performed.

Fig. 6-4. Interview form.

patient that this will be a friendly visit, since eye level contact is almost always more relaxing than the usual nurse-patient (standing-lying) contact. Using a prepared guide, the nurse begins her interview. Fig. 6-4 is a sample interview guide sheet. Each section is considered in whichever sequence the nurse desires. Sometimes the patient will set the sequence of the interview by the questions he asks. The only important aspect of the interview sheet is that all of the pertinent data are covered.

Items for discussion are those relating to the patient's self-image. These might be related to the wearing of dentures, contact lens, or hair pieces. Operating room personnel must be aware of these sometimes nondiscernible items that patients often refuse to part with and will wear into the operating room. In these cases nurses must be careful that they do not cause an injury to the patient or that the items do not become lost or damaged.

Problem areas should be explored. The nurse may ask: Has he had any previous surgery? Has he had any major accidents? With such questions, many times the nurse is able to elicit information that the patient did not mention to his physician. Such information may provide knowledge of problems that need special monitoring in the operating room.

During the interview the nurse should be able to ascertain the patient's command and comprehension of the language. Does he understand what is being said? If not, is an interpreter available to help with the interview? Does he wear a hearing aid? If so, he probably will not be wearing it to surgery. Operating room nurses should be aware of this problem so that they can interact with the patient in a way he can understand.

Family relationships should be explored. Identify those relatives closest to the patient and assess the patient's need to have them near him. If the family is present at the interview, the nurse can provide a support system for them by answering questions they may have. She can escort them to the family waiting area and explain the institution's protocol for dispensing information to families of surgical patients. There may be times when the nurse does not have to lead the interview in determining family relationships. By simply observing the interplay that occurs between the various members, the nurse can make fairly accurate assessments that will determine her own course of action in relation to the patient.

Throughout the interview, the nurse will continually receive impressions of the patient's emotional status. Most of these impressions will come through observation of the patient's behavior in response to her questions. The astute questioner can identify the anxious or fearful patient. Once the emotion has been identified, the nurse can utilize her expertise and knowledge of what happens in surgery to try and allay the patient's fears by substituting knowledge for apprehension of the unknown.

When the nurse has gathered sufficient data and answered the patient's questions, she then begins the preoperative instructions. These include,

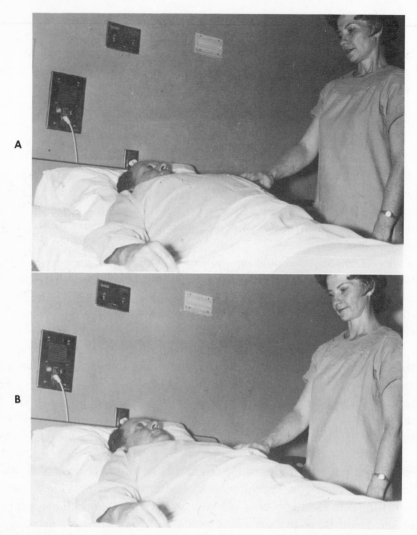

Fig. 6-5. A, The operating room nurse demonstrates the technic for deep breathing and has the patient practice the exercise. **B,** Inspiration is followed by a complete exhalation.

for example, the type of evening meal the patient can expect, the visit from the anesthesiologist, any special procedures that have been ordered preoperatively, such as a Foley catheter or nasogastric tube insertion. If a hypnotic has been ordered, the effect to be expected and the reason for the order should be explained. The reason and importance of an NPO (nothing by mouth) order should be discussed.

Most patients are anxious to follow the physician's orders as they apply to him and, generally speaking, will only violate the rules when they do not understand them. Nurses should be careful to give adequate and meaningful (to the patient) explanations of all events expected to occur.

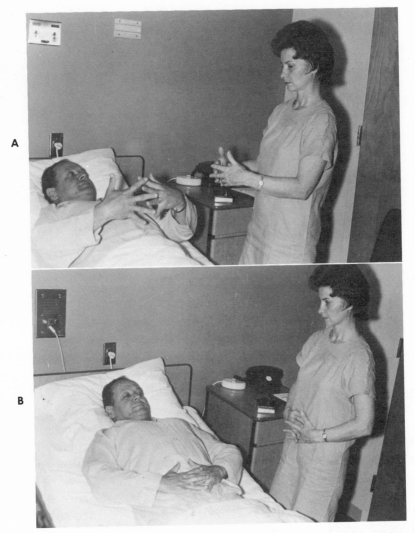

Fig. 6-6. A, The operating room nurse demonstrates the technic of interlacing the fingers together. **B,** The hands are placed across the incisional site to act as a splint when coughing.

The last part of the instructions should cover the postoperative phase, including exercises for the prevention of complications. The patient should be made aware of the importance (to him) and the reasons for following through with the instructions. The best method of ensuring compliance is to make sure the patient understands and can demonstrate each exercise he is expected to perform. In some institutions this teaching can best be done by the unit nurses. The important point is that it *is* done and so validated by both the operating room and unit nurses.

Deep breathing and coughing are vitally important to good respiratory recovery after an inhalation anesthetic. It is probably the most difficult

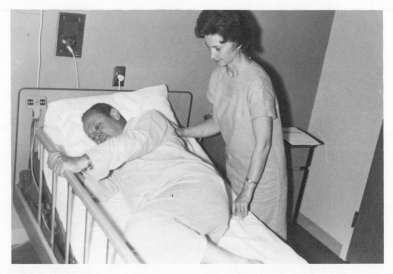

Fig. 6-7. The patient is shown how to turn from side to side in bed using the side rail for leverage.

exercise for the patient who has had an abdominal or thoracic incision. The nurse first demonstrates the technic of deep breathing by inhaling through the nose, letting the abdomen distend, then exhaling through the mouth, pulling the abdomen in until all air has been expelled (Fig. 6-5). The patient should be able to demonstrate the technic to both his own and the nurse's satisfaction. He is then instructed to practice 5 minutes out of each hour for the remainder of the evening and again prior to surgery.

The nurse then demonstrates how the patient can deep breathe and cough without too much discomfort if he has an abdominal incision. A brace or splint is formed by lacing the fingers together and pressing the hands against the site of the incision or by holding a pillow tightly against the abdomen. The effect of the brace is to decrease the discomfort produced by coughing (Fig. 6-6). Emphasis is placed on the danger of complications, such as pneumonia, unless the accumulated gases and secretions are removed quickly and continuously during the postoperative period.

Exercises to prevent venous stasis and thrombophlebitis with an accompanying pulmonary embolus are explained as follows: the patient moves from side to side, bends the knees and brings them up to the chest, then extends the legs toward the foot of the bed (Fig. 6-7 and 6-8). These exercises should be performed every hour until the patient begins to ambulate. Additional exercises such as the flexion, extension, and rotation (internal and external) of the feet (Fig. 6-9) are also beneficial to patients who find it difficult to do other forms of exercise.

At the completion of the interview, the nurse should let the patient

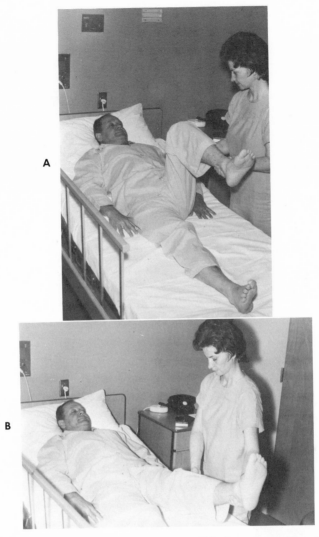

Fig. 6-8. Flexion and extension of the legs. With demonstration, the nurse explains the importance and the "why's" of postsurgical exercises.

know that she will see him when he comes to the operating room, if this is possible. Otherwise she should inform him that other nurses will be caring for him. She will assure him that she will come back to see him in 2 or 3 days after his surgery, if this is possible.

Before leaving the unit, the operating room nurse consults with the unit nursing team and, together, they plan the course of nursing care for the patient (Fig. 6-10). Areas of concern are discussed with the unit nurses who can, in turn, follow through at a team conference to ensure continuity of care.

After charting the visit and noting any observations pertinent to the

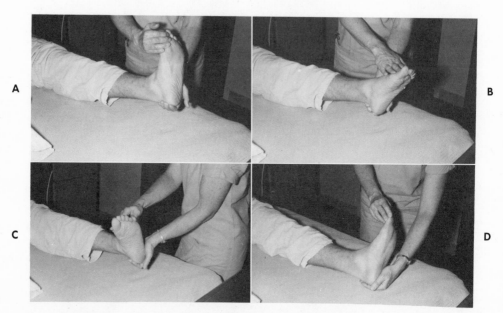

Fig. 6-9. Foot exercises. **A,** Flexion; **B,** extension; **C,** internal rotation; **D,** external rotation.

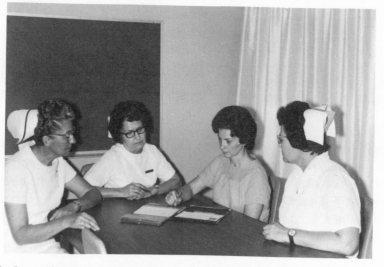

Fig. 6-10. Operating room nurse discusses findings with unit nursing team. An exchange of information concerning the patient is vitally important prior to the patient's arrival in the surgical suite.

surgery, the nurse goes on to complete the rest of the visits for the day. The completed interview sheet is returned to the operating room where, time permitting, it is discussed with the nursing staff. If there is no time for discussion, it can be posted on the bulletin board where the nurses assigned to each room can retrieve it for review before the patient arrives.

A preoperative interview usually takes between 20 and 30 minutes. Prolonged visits seldom benefit the patient. The nurse should be careful not to digress from the purpose of the visit. This does not imply that a carefully rehearsed speech must be adhered to. On the contrary, nurses interviewing patients will discover a variety of personality types. The nurse never knows how the interview will turn out; therefore, she must be prepared to fit her visit and the tone of the interview to the mood of the patient. Memorized speeches will not be effective. Until the nurse learns to establish a friendly, relaxed and interested (in the patient) atmosphere, the patient will sense any insincerity and she will lose him as an audience before the interview begins.

REFERENCES

1. Robinson, L.: Psychological aspects of the care of hospitalized patients, Philadelphia, 1968, F. A. Davis Co., Chapter 3.
2. Ujhely, G. B.: What is realistic emotional support? Am. J. Nurs. 68:758-762, April 1968.
3. Clemons, B.: The operating room nurse in the patient care circuit, Am. J. Nurs. 68:2141-2145, Oct. 1968.
4. Ellison, D.: Patient centered care in the operating room, Nurs. Clin. North Am. 3(4):631-639, Dec. 1968.
5. Adriani, J., editor: Appraisal of current concepts in anesthesiology, vol. 4, St. Louis, 1968, The C. V. Mosby Co., pp. 1-9.
6. Tantum, K. R., and Dripps, R. D.: The scope and challenge of modern anesthesia, Nurs. Clin. North Am. 3(4):591-592, Dec. 1968.

SUGGESTED READINGS

Alexander, C., Schrader, E., and Kneedler, J.: Preoperative visits: The OR nurse unmasks, AORN J. 19:401-412, Feb. 1974.
Ayers, C., and Walton, L.: A guide for the preoperative visit, AORN J. 19:413-418, Feb. 1974.
Bruegel, M. A.: Relationship of preoperative anxiety to perception of postoperative pain, Nurs. Res. 20:26-31, Jan.-Feb. 1971.
Burkhardt, M.: Response to anxiety, Am. J. Nurs. 69:2153-2154, Oct. 1969.
Carnevali, D. L.: Preoperative anxiety, Am. J. Nurs. 66:1536-1538, July 1966.
Clemons, B.: The OR nurse in the patient care circuit, Am. J. Nurs. 68:2141-2145, Oct. 1968.
Depee, J. K.: A critical time for preoperative patients. In Effective therapeutic communication in nursing, monograph 8, ANA Clinical Sessions, New York, 1964, American Nurses' Association, pp. 17-26.
Dumas, R. G.: Psychological preparation for surgery, Am. J. Nurs. 63:52-55, Aug. 1963.
Dumas, R. G., Anderson, B. J., and Leonard, R. C.: The importance of the expressive function in preoperative preparation. In Skipper, J. K., Jr., and Leonard, R. C., editors: Social interaction and patient care, Philadelphia, 1965, J. B. Lippincott Co., pp. 16-29.
Edwards, B.: Preop home visits: Patient perception and nurse self-image, AORN J. 19:419-422, Feb. 1974.
Egbert, L. D.: Psychological support for surgical patients. In Abrams, H. S., editor:

Psychological aspects of surgery; International psychiatry clinics, Boston, 1967, Little, Brown and Co., pp. 37-51.

Fernsebner, W.: Preop visits for eye patients, AORN J. 20:980-985, Dec. 1974.

Field, L. W.: Identifying the psychological aspects of the surgical patient, AORN J. 17:86-90, Jan. 1973.

Healy, K. M.: Does preoperative instruction make a difference? Am. J. Nurs. 68:62-67, Jan. 1968.

Lindeman, C. A.: Nursing intervention with the presurgical patient—Effectiveness and efficiency of group and individual preoperative teaching—Phase two, Nurs. Res. 21:196-209, May-June 1972.

Lindeman, C. A.: Study evaluates effects of preoperative visits, AORN J. 19:427-438, Feb. 1974.

Lindeman, C. A., and Van Aernam, B.: Nursing intervention with the presurgical patient—The effects of structured and unstructured preoperative teaching, Nurs. Res. 20:319-332, July-Aug. 1971.

Mehaffy, N.: Don't just talk about it, Do it, AORN J. 14:81-83, July 1971.

Mezzanotte, E. J.: Group instruction in preparation for surgery, Am. J. Nurs. 70:89-91, Jan. 1970.

Morrison, P. T.: Group visits help T and A patients, AORN J. 20:323-326, Aug. 1974.

Petrillo, M.: Preventing hospital trauma in pediatric patients, Am. J. Nurs. 68:1469-1473, July 1968.

Ridgeway, M.: Preop interviews assure quality care, AORN J. 24:1083-1085, Dec. 1976.

Shetler, M. G.: Operating room nurses go visiting, Am. J. Nurs. 72:1266-1269, July 1972.

Stetzer, S.: Preoperative visits meet patient's tangible needs, AORN J. 19:441-448, Feb. 1974.

Winslow, E., and Fuhs, M. F.: Preoperative assessment for postoperative evaluation, Am. J. Nurs. 73:1372-1374, Aug. 1973.

CHAPTER 7

NURSING CARE IN THE OPERATING ROOM

Nursing care in the operating room presents a multifaceted challenge. Here the nurse has opportunities to prepare the patient for anesthesia, comfort the patient, and use *nursing judgment* in assuring that a safe, efficient surgical procedure takes place.

The nurse is the overseer of the total operating room environment. The information about the patient that was gained in the preoperative visit will be used in the operating room to provide for the patient's safety in positioning and throughout the entire procedure. The patient is constantly observed. The nurse assists in observing skin color, blood loss, and any deviation in alignment of the patient; she is alert to any developing pressure areas on the patient's body and is prepared for emergencies. The operating room personnel substitute for the "conscious" activities of the unconscious patient.

Whether scrubbing, circulating, or supervising, the operating room nurse is always aware of the patient's total environment. The *patient* is the foremost concern. The nurse's orientation is twofold: technical and psychosocial. The operating room nurse can make beginning assessments of how the *psychologic* and *physiologic trauma* of surgery is affecting the *whole patient* (certainly a fertile area for nursing research).

As overseer of the surgical environment, the operating room nurse also coordinates efforts of other team members and teaches them. As stated previously, the registered nurse will most likely be the circulating nurse during an operation. If a less-prepared team member is in the scrub role, the nurse will supervise and teach. Above all, the nurse constantly *observes*.

It is impossible to overstress communications in the operating suite. Especially important is the communication between nurse and surgeon in each room. Together, as colleagues, they plan actions that ensure safety. They confer on special equipment or positioning needed, on expectations of what will be found during the procedure, and on expected deviations from routines. They continue to communicate, sometimes nonverbally as well as verbally, throughout the operation.

The surgeon, nurse, and anesthesiologist can share their respective assessments of the patient so that all findings are known and subsequent actions planned. The patient may have shared pertinent information with one professional person and not another. All members must feel that they are vital to team functioning and have something to contribute. Information sharing, before and during the procedure, aids this goal. It is mandatory that a tone of respect and consideration prevail, so that the team can function smoothly and efficiently and that the progress of the operation not be hindered.

The operating room nurse is sensitive to minute changes in the patient's condition. The nurse notes technics and procedures being carried out and must be sure that the patient is undergoing surgery in an optimal environment. Basic knowledge in applied psychology and psychophysiology gives the operating room nurse this prerogative. Nursing judgment is essential to the patient and the other members of this surgical team.

During the operation the nurse must be aware of principles of various components of the surgery. Among these are asepsis (Chapter 5), patient positioning, instrumentation, and scrubbing, gowning, and gloving. This chapter emphasizes these and other principles. Details of each operative procedure, names of instruments, and surgeon's preferences are left to the individual institution. Only the essentials are dealt with here.

ADMISSION OF THE PATIENT TO THE OPERATING ROOM

Mental preparation of the patient is as important as physical preparation. This is often overlooked when preparing and admitting the patient to surgery. Fear of the unknown, separation from family members, and fear of the results or the outcome of a procedure may cause complications. Preoperative visits by operating room and postanesthesia personnel, as discussed in Chapter 6, can help to relieve these fears.

The nurse must avoid unnecessary exposure of the patient. The patient should be given an explanation of what is being done in preparation and why it is being done. Occasionally a delay is necessary. In this case, an explanation should be given to the patient and his waiting family.

It is much easier to calm a crying, frightened child if he is allowed to have his very own "security blanket" or a favorite toy with him. The nurse must be sure that this trusted "friend" is returned safely with the patient to his unit.

When the patient arrives in the operating room, the nurse first introduces herself. At this point, it is most important to identify the patient by asking his name and checking his name band with the chart. Correct identification is the responsibility of every member of the team who has contact with the patient.

In addition to carefully identifying the patient, the admitting operating room nurse is also responsible for checking the chart. Most hospitals have

Yes   No

____ ____ Surgery consent signed

____ ____ Special consents signed
____ ____   Incomplete abortion
____ ____   Sterilization
____ ____   Disposal of amputated limb

____ ____ History and physical in chart

____ ____ Laboratory reports in chart

____ ____ Allergies

____ ____ Preoperative medication given and charted

____ ____ TPR charted

____ ____ Identification band legible and in proper place

____ ____ Identification plate on chart

____ ____ Voided—Time _____

____ ____ Underclothing removed

____ ____ Jewelry removed (wedding rings may be taped or secured)

____ ____ Contact lenses removed

____ ____ Dentures and partial plates removed

____ ____ Hairpins, clips removed

____ ____ Other prostheses removed _____

____ ____ Presence of metal implants

____ ____ Makeup removed

____ ____ Family instructed where to wait

____ ____ Special toy or blanket with child

____ ____   Name or article _____

____ ____ Old records with chart

____ ____ Preoperative teaching done and charted

____ ____ Shave prep done

_____
Signature of nurse releasing patient

Fig. 7-1. Preoperative check list.

an admission procedure and a preoperative check list (Fig. 7-1). The check list is used by the unit nurse in patient preparation, but this is again verified by the operating room nurse.

When admitting the patient to the operating room, the following must be checked:

I. Patient name on chart, operative schedule, and identification band.

II. Operative permit. This must be properly signed, dated, and witnessed. The procedure listed on the permit must agree with the operating room schedule. States and hospitals vary in their requirements as to who may sign a consent. In general, the following rules apply:

A. An adult who is responsible for his own actions and not under narcosis may sign his own consent. It should be signed by writing his name in full. A married woman should use her given name, not her husband's.

B. A parent or guardian must sign the permit for a minor. Any married minor or one who is earning his own living may sign for himself. Also, a pregnant minor may sign for any procedure having to do with her pregnancy.

C. Some procedures require special consents and consultations. Therapeutic abortions, sterilizations, and primary cesarean sections are among these procedures.

III. History and physical examination record. This should be on the chart before the anesthesiologist sees the patient preoperatively but must be completed before the surgery begins.

IV. Laboratory reports. Each hospital has a minimum number of laboratory analyses that must be done and reported before surgery. The operating room nurse should see that the necessary reports are on the chart.

V. Prostheses, implants, dentures, jewelry, artificial hair or eyelashes, contact lenses, and objects in the mouth. In a child it is wise to check for gum or candy in the mouth.

VI. Surgical shave and preparation of the operative site.

VII. Preoperative medication; when given, any signs of side or adverse effects. The nurse should especially watch for symptoms of perspiration, weakness, dizziness, or rapid pulse rate.

A premedicated patient should never be left alone. A calm, reassuring operating room nurse can do much to help the patient at this time. Also, a sleepy, quiet patient may forget he is on a narrow stretcher and fall in spite of the straps. Thus, for reasons of both comfort and safety, the nurse must constantly attend the medicated patient. Conversation and noise must be kept to a minimum; a few softly spoken words usually are adequate. The *presence* of a nurse is the crucial point. Especially to be avoided at this time are conversations among the personnel about other patients; these are frequently misinterpreted by the patient and must be avoided. The nurse must remember at all times that the patient is an individual and not a "case."

The patient is moved into the operating room and placed on the operating room table (Fig. 7-2).

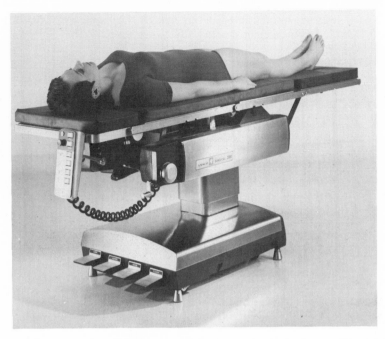

Fig. 7-2. An operating room table on which the patient can be positioned for any surgical procedure. (Courtesy American Sterilizer Company, Erie, Pennsylvania.)

SCRUBBING, GOWNING, AND GLOVING

The purpose of the scrubbing done by the team members is to render their skin *surgically clean* by reducing the number of organisms on the skin to a minimum. Team members are clad in scrub suits or dresses, caps that cover *all* of the hair, and masks that are positioned snugly and comfortably, completely covering the nose and mouth.

Procedures for the hand and arm scrub will vary from hospital to hospital. Some will use an anatomic scrub, whereas others will use the time-measured scrub. Various chemical agents are used for the skin scrub; most, however, will have either a hexachlorophene or an iodine base. Regardless of the procedure or chemical agent used, certain principles must be followed:

1. Nails should be short, clean, and free of nail polish.
2. Light friction is sufficient. Heavy friction can cause the dermis to bleed or "weep."
3. A different sterile brush or scrub sponge may be used for each hand; many disposable brushes and sponges are on the market.
4. The nails should be cleaned with a sterile or disinfected nail cleaner made of stainless steel or plastic.
5. Hands should always be held above elbow level so that drippings run from a clean to an unclean area.
6. Arms must be kept well away from the body.

7. Every person should scrub between all procedures, whether the procedure is clean or contaminated. Even though the hands or arms have not become contaminated, it is necessary to remove bacteria that have multiplied under the gloves.
8. The surgical scrub must be a concentrated effort. Time must be watched or strokes counted.

Procedure for the timed scrub

1. Wet the hands and arms and apply a small amount of the chemical agent. Wash the hands and arms without a brush. Clean the nails and rinse well.
2. Take a brush or sponge, apply a small amount of soap and scrub each area the prescribed amount of time (usually about 2 minutes), starting with the nails and proceeding to the fingers, hands, and arms to 1 to 2 inches above the elbows. Add small amounts of water or chemical agent as needed.
3. Repeat on the opposite arm, using a new sterile brush or sponge.
4. Rinse well, keeping hands higher than elbows.

Procedure for the anatomic scrub

1. Same as timed scrub.
2. Starting with the nails, scrub the prescribed number of strokes, usually 25 strokes to the nails and fingers and 15 to the hands and arms.
3. Repeat on the opposite arm, using a new sterile brush or sponge.
4. Rinse well, keeping hands higher than elbows.

Procedure for the one-brush/sponge scrub

1. Same as timed scrub (Concurrent movement on both arms and hands, proceeding up to elbows).
2. Take a brush or sponge, apply a small amount of soap or lather, and scrub both hands for the prescribed amount of time (usually 2 minutes on each hand).
3. Scrub both arms to 1 to 2 inches above the elbows.
4. Rinse well, keeping hands higher than elbows.

The purpose of sterile gown and gloves is to cover the unsterile scrub suit or dress and the surgically clean hands and arms in order to prevent contamination of the wound and supplies.

Procedure for gowning

1. The towel is grasped by one corner, permitting it to unfold. Bending slightly forward from the waist will help to prevent contamination of the lower end of the towel from the clothing.
2. One hand is dried starting from the fingers and working up to the elbow (Fig. 7-3, *A*).
3. With the dried hand, grasp the lower end of the towel, dry the fingers of the second hand, and work up to the elbow.
4. Care must be taken to prevent contamination of the towel and hands.
5. Discard the towel.
6. Grasp the sterile gown at the neckline, hold it away from the body and allow it to unfold with the inside of the gown toward the wearer (Fig. 7-3, *B*).
7. Slip the hands into the sleeves with the hands held upward.
8. The circulating nurse then reaches inside the gown, pulling the inside sleeve seam (Fig. 7-3, *C*).
9. The circulating nurse ties the back of the gown, touching only the ties and

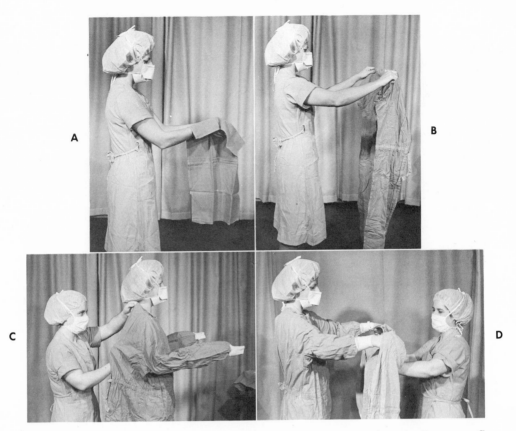

Fig. 7-3. Gowning. **A,** Drying the hand; **B,** grasping and opening sterile gown; **C,** circulating nurse assists in gowning; **D,** scrub nurse assists other personnel to gown.

outer edges of the gown. When tying the waist ties, it is helpful in pre-venting contamination if the scrubbed person bends slightly in the direc-tion that will bring the ties away from the sterile gown.

10. After the scrub nurse is gowned and gloved, she will assist other scrub personnel to gown. In so doing, she cuffs the sterile gown over her hands so as not to contaminate herself (Fig. 7-3, *D*).

Gloving

Two methods of gloving are used—the closed method and the open method. The closed method is preferred because there is less chance of con-tamination of the outside of the sterile gloves by the surgically clean hands. However, if a glove must be replaced during the procedure, the open method of gloving is used.

Procedure for closed gloving

1. The hands are only brought through to the cuffs of the gown: the cuffs must cover both hands so that cuff edges have not been touched by the bare hands.
2. Pick up the first glove by the folded cuff with the hand covered by the cuff of the gown. This is usually done with the left hand (Fig. 7-4, *A*).

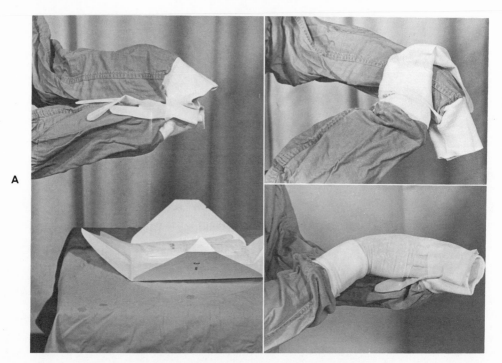

Fig. 7-4. Closed gloving. **A,** Picking up the first glove with the cuffed hand; **B,** pulling glove over cuff of gown; **C,** putting on second glove.

3. Place the glove, palm and thumb side down, on the forearm of the opposite hand.
4. Pull the glove cuff over the knitted cuff so that it completely covers the cuff (Fig. 7-4, *B*).
5. Work fingers into the glove and pull the glove onto the hand using the covered hand.
6. Repeat this process with the opposite hand (Fig. 7-4, *C*).

Procedure for open gloving

1. When gowning, the hands are brought all the way through the cuffs of the gown. After gowning, pick up one glove by its cuff (Fig. 7-5, *A*); either hand may be used. Pull the glove onto the opposite hand using the cuff and being careful not to touch any other part of the glove (Fig. 7-5, *B*).
2. With the gloved hand, slide the fingers (excluding thumb) inside the cuff of the second glove (Fig. 7-5, *C*). Pull the glove onto the hand and the cuff of the glove over the cuff of the gown. Caution must be taken to avoid inward rolling of the glove cuff as it is being brought up on the hand; this would contaminate the outside of the glove from the surgically clean hand.
3. Draw the cuff of the opposite glove over the gown cuff.

ANESTHESIA

The choice of anesthesia is made by the surgeon and the anesthesiologist. The type of anesthesia will depend on the patient's condition, age, any

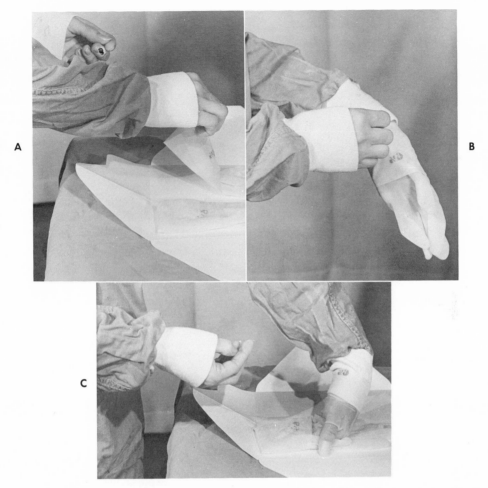

Fig. 7-5. Open gloving. A, Picking up first glove; B, pulling glove onto hand; C, sliding gloved fingers inside cuff of second glove.

medication he has been taking, the surgical procedure, duration of the procedure, idiosyncrasy for drugs, and the patient's preference.

Induction

The operating room nurse (usually the circulating nurse) has definite responsibilities during the induction phase of anesthesia. The nurse must not leave the room at this time and should be near the patient to assist the anesthesiologist and to provide comfort and security to the patient. Children may need to be restrained during this time, but only if absolutely necessary. The nurse should avoid touching or moving the patient during the induction until the anesthesiologist gives his approval. The nurse may place her hand over the patient without touching him and, in this way, provide protection should the patient move excessively or become excited.

If a knee strap is applied before the anesthesia, the patient may be quietly told that it is to protect him on a narrow table.

The room should be quiet during induction and doors should be closed. As the patient is anesthetized, the last sense to be lost is hearing; slight noises may seem exaggerated and very loud to the patient. Caution must be exerted in any conversation that goes on at this time. Stimulation to the patient is to be avoided for it could cause laryngospasm, vomiting, or excitement.

Types of anesthesia

Anesthesia is the partial or complete loss of sensation with or without the loss of consciousness. Anesthesia may be general, regional, or local. An analgesic, on the other hand, is an agent that relieves pain.

General anesthesia. General anesthetics block the awareness centers of the brain. When an adequate amount of the anesthetic agent has reached the brain, the patient becomes unconscious. General anesthetic agents may

Table 2. The four stages of anesthesia

	From	*To*	*Patient status*	*Nurse should*
Stage I	Beginning administration of gas or drug	Loss of consciousness	May appear inebriated, drowsy, dizzy	Close OR doors. Keep room quiet. Stand by patient to assist, if necessary
Stage II	Loss of consciousness	Relaxation	May appear excited; may breathe irregularly; may move arms and legs or body. Patient very susceptible to external stimuli (noise, being touched suddenly)	Be ready to restrain patient if needed. Remain at patient's side, quiet and alert. Assist anesthesiologist, if needed
Stage III	(Surgical anesthesia stage) relaxation	Loss of reflexes; depression of vital functions	Regular respiration, contracted pupils, eyelid reflexes disappear, jaw relaxed. Auditory sensation lost during Stage III	Begin prep only when anesthesiologist indicates Stage III reached and patient is under good control
Stage IV	(Danger stage) Vital functions too depressed	Respiratory failure; possible cardiac arrest	Not breathing. Little or no heartbeat or pulse	If arrest occurs, react immediately to assist in establishing airway. Provide cardiac arrest tray, drugs, syringes, long needles. Assist surgeon with closed or open cardiac massage

From Nursing care of the patient in OB-GYN surgery, Somerville, New Jersey, 1966, Ethicon, Inc. (Reproduced with permission.)

be administered by inhalation, intravenously, or rectally. The method used will depend on the patient, the procedure, and the position of the patient.

General anesthesia is usually a combination of drugs and gases. A common fast-acting induction agent, given primarily for the patient's comfort, is sodium pentothal. A mask is then applied, and a mixture of oxygen and anesthetic gases (nitrous oxide, halothane, or others) is administered. Depending on the need for relaxation, narcotics, muscle relaxants, or both may be administered intravenously during the procedure.

The four stages of anesthesia are described in Table 2. It is vital that the operating room nurse be familiar with these and be able to recognize all four phases.

Open drop administration. In the open drop administration a volatile liquid anesthetic is dropped onto a gauze-covered mask and the patient inhales the vapor. Supplementary oxygen may be given by nasal catheter. The vapor is irritating and drying to mucous membranes and skin. The eyes and skin must be protected. The disadvantages are that high concentrations of explosive gases are present in the room and there is no control of respirations. Examples of agents utilized in the open drop method are ether and vinethene.

Administration by mask. Vapors from liquids or gases under pressure in tanks are administered in a combination through a tube and mask. Regulated amounts are passed into a mixing chamber and then into a rubber rebreathing bag. These may be administered by either the open, semiclosed, or closed method.

In the *open method* the patient inhales only anesthetic agents and oxygen delivered from the anesthesia machine; he exhales through a valve directly into the atmosphere. In the *semiclosed method*, the patient rebreathes a portion of the exhaled gases and the remainder goes into the surrounding atmosphere through an escape valve. In the *closed method* the anesthetic gases flow directly into the patient's lung either by mask or endotracheal tube. Soda lime in a cannister removes exhaled carbon dioxide. With this method of administration there is no escape of gas into the environment. There is also complete control of inhaled gases; little agent escapes into the atmosphere. This is the safest method to use with explosive gases.

An *endotracheal tube* is usually used in the closed method. The tube is inserted into the tracheobronchial tree by blind or direct laryngoscopy. The balloon at the end of the tube is inflated to ensure a snug fit and to prevent leakage of gases and air (Fig. 7-6). This gives total control of inhaled gases and complete control over the patient's respirations. An endotracheal tube is sometimes necessary also because of the location of the surgery (tonsillectomy) or because of the position of the patient (prone). In these instances, use of a mask would not be physically possible.

Intravenous administration. Occasionally an anesthetic agent is given intravenously. Some barbiturate agents, such as sodium pentothal, are used

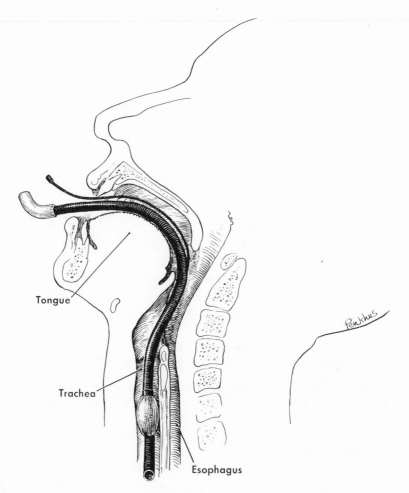

Fig. 7-6. Placement of endotracheal tube for administration of anesthesia (note inflation of cuff).

as basal anesthesia and may be given intravenously for induction of the patient.

Local anesthesia. In local, or regional, anesthesia a drug injected into a specified area interrupts the normal passage of sensory impulses to a certain area or region.

Nurses monitoring patients under local anesthesia should have a nursing history available—one that points up potential patient problems. This history should include past respiratory problems, smoking habits, shortness of breath, and presence of cough. Oxygen should never exceed 5 to 6 liters/minute for patients with chronic respiratory problems. Hypoxia in these patients stimulates the respiratory drive. A high percentage of oxygen may depress respirations.

Topical administration. The drug is applied directly to the surface of

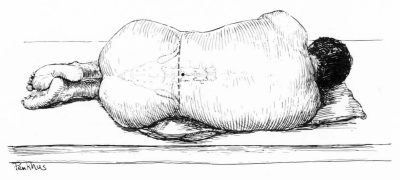

Penthus

Fig. 7-7. Position for administration of spinal anesthesia. Needle is inserted between L-$_3$ and L-$_4$, and the drug is injected into the subarachnoid space. Patient is in lateral position with knees and hips flexed and head down to help widen the interspinous spaces and facilitate needle insertion.

an involved area. It is usually used for anesthesia of the respiratory passages.

Local infiltration. This method involves a drug injected into the tissues surrounding the incisional area.

Nerve block. In this method a drug is injected into and around a nerve or bundle of nerves. Nerve blocks are used not only for surgical procedures but also to ascertain the cause of pain, to relieve pain following amputation, and to decrease neuralgic pain and increase circulation in certain vascular diseases.

Spinal administration. In spinal administration the drug is injected into the subarachnoid space causing anesthesia and muscle relaxation below the point of injection. Fig. 7-7 illustrates the position of the patient for administration of spinal anesthesia.

Caudal administration. A drug is injected into the caudal canal epidurally. This produces anesthesia of the perineum.

Regional, or local, anesthetics have many advantages, such as use in emergency procedures when the patient has eaten, for alcoholics who require large amounts of general anesthesia, and in childbirth since they have no effect on the fetus. In local anesthesia the patient is awake and conscious and is able to cooperate with the surgeon during the procedure. Often the progress of the operation is determined by patient responses and answers to questions. Local anesthetics do not irritate the respiratory system.

Some disadvantages of local anesthetics are: (1) there is no control over the drug once it is injected; (2) respirations may be depressed because of paralysis of intercostal muscles; (3) hypotension may result; and (4) there may be headache caused by loss of spinal fluid. In addition, the patient may suffer from psychic strain since he is awake during the pro-

Table 3. Agents used in anesthesia administration

Agent	Administration	Induction	Advantages	Disadvantages	Nursing precautions
Halothane (Fluothane)	Inhalation	Rapid and smooth	Nonflammable Pleasant odor Nonirritating Little excitement Rapid emergence Seldom causes nausea or vomiting	Requires special vaporizer Narrow margin of safety May depress cardiovascular system Limited relaxation Expensive May cause liver damage	Watch for bradycardia and hypotension Use of epinephrine, with this agent, may cause cardiac arrhythmias, including ventricular fibrillation
Nitrous oxide	Inhalation	Rapid	Rapid induction and recovery Nonflammable Few aftereffects	Poor relaxation May produce hypoxia Except for short procedures, must be used with other agents	When used with other agents, follow those precautions
Vinyl ether (Vinethene)	Open drop Inhalation	Rapid	Good for short procedures Good relaxation Small incidence of excitement	May cause kidney and liver damage Great danger of overdose Irritating Flammable and explosive Irritating to skin	Protect skin and eyes Practice explosion safeguards
Penthrane	Inhalation	Slow	Nonflammable and nonexplosive Excellent muscle relaxation Seldom causes nausea or vomiting	Requires special vaporizer and skillful administration May cause kidney or liver damage	Long postoperative depressant action Patient requires close observation
Enflurane (Ethrane)	Inhalation	Rapid and smooth	Nonflammable Nonirritating to respiratory tract Good muscle relaxant Eliminated rapidly	Not compatible with epinephrine Requires special vaporizer	Administration with epinephrine may cause ventricular fibrillation Body temperature may fall and patient may shiver following prolonged use Watch for hypotension, respiratory depression, arrhythmias, nausea, and vomiting

Isoflurane (Forane)	Inhalation	Rapid	Nonflammable Rapid recovery Cardiac output remains stable Good muscle relaxant No evidence of renal or hepatic damage	Requires special vaporizer May be irritating to respiratory tract during induction	Watch for nausea, vomiting, excitement, and shivering
Ether	Open drop Inhalation	Slow	Good relaxation and wide margin of safety Inexpensive Nontoxic	Long recovery (elimination may take 8 hours) Unpleasant odor Irritating to skin, mucous membranes, lungs, and kidneys Causes nausea and vomiting, urinary retention, and acidosis Explosive and flammable	Protect skin and eyes Expect nausea and vomiting Prevent aspiration Practice explosion safeguards
Cyclopropane	Inhalation	Rapid and pleasant	Rapid induction and emergence Wide margin of safety Good relaxation Well tolerated	Explosive May cause cardiac arrhythmias, shock, bronchospasm, and acidosis	Use explosion safeguards Observe blood pressure
Ketamine (Ketalar)	Intravenous Intramuscular	Rapid	Short action Excellent for diagnostic and short, topical surgical procedures May be used to supplement weaker agents such as nitrous oxide	Too rapid administration causes respiratory depression Induces blood pressure rise May produce dreams or hallucinations Patients may act irrationally when emerging from anesthesia	Avoid stimulation of patient by touching or talking Resuscitative equipment must be available
Thiopental sodium (Pentothal Sodium)	Intravenous Rectal	Rapid and pleasant	Rapid, pleasant induction and recovery (patient has no recollection of mask) Nonirritating; nonflammable Easy administration Good for short procedures and hypnosis during regional anesthesia	Large doses cause respiratory-circulatory depression Wide variation in tolerance Poor relaxation	Watch for respiratory and circulatory depression Be prepared for possible laryngospasm

Continued.

Table 3. Agents used in anesthesia administration—cont'd

Agent	Administration	Induction	Advantages	Disadvantages	Nursing precautions
Innovar (combination of inapsine and sublimaze)	Intramuscular Intravenous	Rapid	Produces a state of quiescence with decreased motor activity and decreased responsiveness to painful stimuli Patient is unresponsive to auditory stimuli but does not lose consciousness Good premedication for anesthesia	Should not be given in combination with hypnotics or strong analgesics May cause respiratory depression, apnea, laryngospasm, bronchospasm, and hallucinations	Observe for respiratory depression, cardiac arrhythmias
Fentanyl (Sublimaze)	Intramuscular Intravenous	Rapid	Rapid induction 80 to 100 times more potent than morphine Duration of action shorter than morphine or meperidine	Degree of respiratory depression may be greater than morphine May cause respiratory depression, nausea, vomiting, bradycardia, muscular rigidity	Observe for muscular rigidity and respiratory depression Doses of narcotics should be reduced by ¼ to ⅓ of usual dose
Lidocaine hydrochloride (Xylocaine)	Infiltration Topical Block or spinal	Rapid	Action is more rapid, more intense, and longer acting than procaine Is a local vasodilator Used to treat arrhythmias during heart surgery or general anesthesia; suppresses laryngeal or pharyngeal reflexes	Few; well tolerated Untoward effects may occur from allergy, overdose, or faulty injection	Initial effect of overdose is depression rather than excitement Watch for drowsiness, respiratory arrest, cardiovascular collapse, and cardiac arrest
Procaine hydrochloride (Novocaine; Ethocaine)	Subcutaneous Intramuscular Intravenous Spinal	Rapid	Low toxicity Good duration of action Inexpensive	Possible idiosyncrasy Slow action	May involve central nervous and cardiovascular systems; watch for reaction; hypotension, bradycardia, thready pulse, shock
Cocaine	Topical	Rapid	Rapid action Patient is conscious	Abolishes throat reflexes when applied in this area High toxicity May be fatal if injected	Watch for cocaine reaction: excitement, restlessness, confusion, hypertension, tachycardia, rapid shallow respirations

cedure. Consideration must also be given to the possibility of infection if poor technic is used in administration.

Miscellaneous. Two types of anesthesia that are seldom used but still very beneficial in selected cases are cryothermia and hypnoanesthesia.

Cryothermia. Cryothermia is anesthesia produced by cooling an extremity. The affected limb is packed in an ice pack for 4 to 16 hours at a temperature of from 2° to 8° C. This method is useful in elderly poor-risk patients who require amputation.

Hypnoanesthesia. Selected patients may be hypnotized and rendered free of pain. While this method is still very controversial, it is useful in obstetrics and dental surgery when administered by a skilled and qualified practitioner. Prehypnotic suggestion may be used to alter the postdelivery or postoperative course of a patient. Preoperative suggestions are designed to help the patient eliminate postoperative pain, nausea, and vomiting.

Table 3 is a summary of the agents most commonly used in anesthesia administration.

Scavenging systems

Recent studies reported by a Committee of the American Society of Anesthesiologists point out that operating room personnel are subject to increased health hazards probably caused by exposure to waste anesthesia gases. Spontaneous abortions occur more frequently among women exposed to the operating room environment during the first trimester. The number of congenital abnormalities is increased about 60% in exposed females. In male and female personnel exposed, the rate of cancer, hepatic and renal disease is increased.

Scavenging systems have been devised. One system uses an activated charcoal filter and is effective for halogenated compounds only. Another system utilizes the vacuum. No system is 100% effective, and any system is as effective as the user makes it. Careless spillage of liquid anesthetics and poorly maintained anesthesia equipment will minimize the effectiveness of scavenging systems.

PATIENT POSITIONING

The circulating nurse usually has responsibility for positioning the patient for surgery. However, the surgeon and other team members may supervise and assist.

The optimal position provides maximal safety and comfort for the patient, allows the surgeon an accessible operative area, and allows the anesthesiologist to administer the anesthetic and observe the patient.

Before the surgery begins, the nurse must see that all of the necessary positioning attachments and equipment are in the room. The hospital procedure book and surgeon preference card should be checked for needed equipment. An anesthetized patient must *never* be moved before the anesthesiologist indicates that the patient is ready to be moved and positioned.

It is important that the patient be moved slowly and with no sudden movements. If the patient's legs are to be placed in stirrups, for example, it is important that both legs be raised, positioned, and lowered at the same time. Turning a patient too quickly can cause circulatory depression. The anesthesiologist will usually move the patient's head in order to protect the endotracheal tube and the patient's airway.

Many complications can arise from faulty or careless positioning. One of the most serious is injury to the brachial nerve plexi (located in the axillary area) or the ulnar nerves (located along the inner surfaces of the upper arms). Neuropathies are caused by stretching or compressing nerves. Stretching produces mechanical damage to the nerve trunk. Compression causes ischemia to the nerves and myoneural junction. If ischemia is prolonged (as when a tourniquet is left tightly in place too long), necrosis may occur. Ruptures of intraneural capillaries cause hematomas, which compress surrounding nerve fibers. These fibers may recover or they may become completely necrotic. Abduction of an arm to more than ninety degrees would cause pain in a conscious patient, but this pain would not be felt by the anesthetized patient.

The operating room nurse, then, has responsibilities not only to ensure a beginning optimal position for the patient but also to observe throughout the procedure for pressure points and unprotected bony prominences. Drapes may become heavy over the patient's toes, for example, and team members may change positions during the procedure in such a way that they are exerting pressure on vulnerable parts of the patient's body.

Principles of positioning

Regardless of the surgical procedure or the patient position, there are certain principles of which the nurse must be aware if the patient is to be protected:

1. Dignity of the patient must be maintained. Even when the patient is anesthetized, undue exposure must be avoided. Positioning that is extreme or that may be embarrassing to the patient is usually done after induction of anesthesia.
2. Respiratory exchange must remain unopposed throughout the procedure. The jaw should be forward to maintain a patent airway. Constriction or pressure on the chest must be avoided in order to permit free exchange of gases.
3. Muscles, nerves, and bony prominences must be protected from pressure. Improper positioning or lack of adequate padding can cause permanent damage to nerves. Elbows, shoulders, toes, and fingers are especially prone to pressure damage. Care must be taken to avoid placing a knee strap directly over the knee. Elbow guards and sheets may be used to protect the elbows, arms, and hands.
4. Adequate circulation must be maintained. Pressure on any body part, especially extremities, is to be avoided. Sludging of blood occurs when circulation is poor; this may cause the formation of a thrombus. Surgeons occasionally wrap the legs with elastic bandages or apply antiemboletic stockings to prevent this.

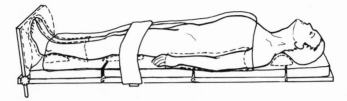

Fig. 7-8. Dorsal position. *1.* Head in line with body. *2.* Arms, palms down, along side of body. *3.* Arms secured under lift sheet (shown in dotted lines). *4.* Padded strap over legs, 2 inches above knees. *5.* Folded towels (shown in dotted lines) are placed under feet, ankles, knees, and neck to maintain slight flexion, optimal venous return, and unobstructed respiratory passage. *6.* Flannel surgical "booties" are shown in dotted lines; these are used to provide additional warmth and to minimize dispersal of foot detritus on the surgical table. *7.* A bath blanket (cotton flannel covering), shown in outline, over the patient for warmth and protection from exposure. Although only indicated in this, the bath blanket is always assumed to cover the surgical patient until ready for the presurgical prep.

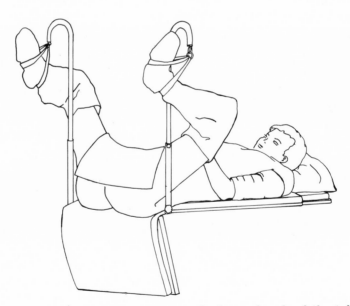

Fig. 7-9. Lithotomy position. *1.* Hips well over the lower break of the table. *2.* Arms crossed over chest and secured under gown. *3.* Both legs are placed into the stirrup slings at the same time (after the patient is anesthetized). Two people are needed to raise patient's legs. Legs are slowly flexed and rotated outward to prevent dislocation. Buttocks should be 1 to 2 inches over the edge of table when lower section of table is dropped. *4.* Pressure on inner lower legs from contact with stirrup poles must be avoided. *5.* Both legs are removed from stirrups at the same time and slowly lowered to table level.

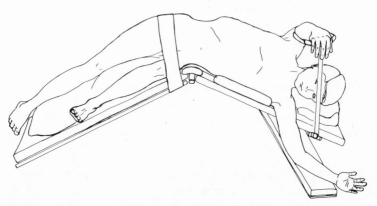

Fig. 7-10. Kidney position. *1.* Patient is on side with body close to edge of table where surgeon will be standing; lumbar region over the kidney rest. *2.* Lower leg is flexed, upper leg straight with pillow between legs. *3.* Arms on double arm board or lower arm on arm board and upper arm extended (may be placed on special arm holder) and with padding between the arms. *4.* Padded knee strap 2 inches above knees. *5.* Padded kidney rest (body elevator) is raised and table flexed. *6.* A wide adhesive tape strip over hips and shoulders, attached to table for support. Upper shoulder, hip, and ankle should be in a straight line. *7.* Rolled towel or foam rubber pad in and under dependent axilla to protect plexus.

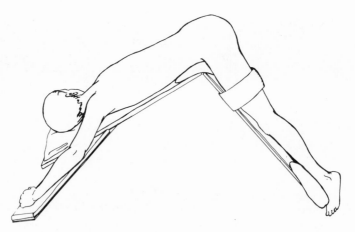

Fig. 7-11. Jackknife or Kraske position. *1.* Patient in prone position with hips over break of table. *2.* Wide armboard under head of mattress to support arms. *3.* Pillow under lower legs and ankles. *4.* Padded knee strap 2 inches above knees. *5.* Table is flexed to an acute angle. *6.* Small towel roll or foam rubber pad under each shoulder to protect plexus.

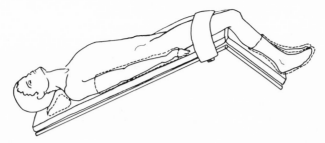

Fig. 7-12. Trendelenburg position. *1.* Patient on back with the knees over the lower break of the table. *2.* Arms, palms down, along side of body. *3.* Padded strap 2 inches above knees. *4.* Head of table lowered. *5.* Knees flexed by lowering the foot section of the surgical table.

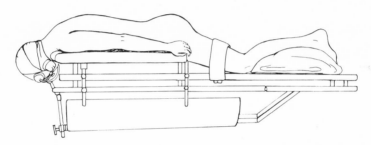

Fig. 7-13. Cerebellar craniotomy (prone) position. *1.* Special head rest must be well padded; face, eyes, ears are protected (in regular prone position, head will be turned to side). *2.* Arms along side of body. *3.* Pillow under lower legs and ankles. *4.* Padded knee strap 2 inches above knees.

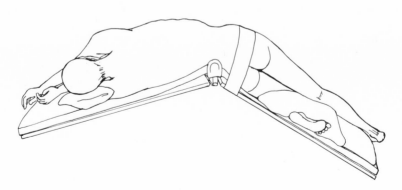

Fig. 7-14. Lateral or chest (thoracotomy) position. *1.* Patient on side with body at edge of table; special support at waist or lower chest region. *2.* Lower leg flexed, upper leg straight with pillow between legs. *3.* Arms outstretched above chest region. *4.* Sandbag along abdomen and chest to prevent the patient from rolling. *5.* Wide adhesive tape strip over the hip and attached to table for support.

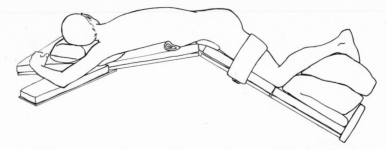

Fig. 7-15. Laminectomy position. *1.* Patient in prone position with lumbar spine over center break of table. *2.* Two large laminectomy rolls (or other firm padding) are placed longitudinally to support the chest, from axilla to hip; additional padding to protect the bony prominences of hips, knees, and feet. *3.* Wide armboard for arm support. *4.* Padded strap 2 inches above knees. *5.* Table is flexed and tilted so that head and upper back are on the same plane.

Figs. 7-8 through 7-15 are examples of the most commonly used positioning methods. An explanation of each accompanies the diagram.

SKIN PREPARATION AND DRAPING

In order to prevent skin bacteria from entering the body, it is important that the skin be properly cleansed. The skin preparation, or "prep," is usually done in two stages.

Stage 1 takes place the night before surgery when the operative site is shaved and cleansed. There are exceptions to this. Some prefer that the shave be done just prior to the surgery. Bacteriologically, the latter is preferred because then the bacteria have less time to proliferate on the skin that has been abraded by the razor. Shaving the operative area ensures cleanliness and prevents hair from being carried into the wound to act as a foreign body or bearer of bacteria.

Prior to shaving the operative area, the nurse should fully explain the procedure to the patient. Since it is necessary to expose parts of the body, every effort should be made to minimize embarrassment to the patient. It is important to act in a considerate, professional manner. While shaving the patient, the nurse has an excellent opportunity to talk with him and answer his questions. Ideally, the shave is done by the same nurse who carries out the preoperative care for the patient.

After shaving the area, the nurse cleanses the skin and inspects it for rashes, lesions, or irritation. Any abnormal skin condition should be reported.

After the patient is anesthetized and positioned in the operating room, stage 2 of skin preparation takes place; the second "prep" is done. The operative site and an extensive area around it are scrubbed with sterile gauze squares or sponges and a chemical agent. The mechanical friction

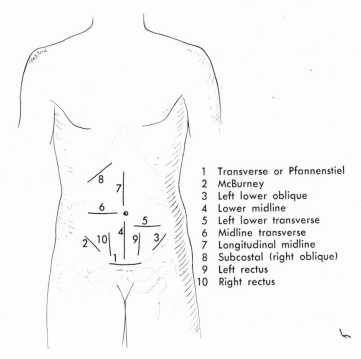

1   Transverse or Pfannenstiel
2   McBurney
3   Left lower oblique
4   Lower midline
5   Left lower transverse
6   Midline transverse
7   Longitudinal midline
8   Subcostal (right oblique)
9   Left rectus
10   Right rectus

Fig. 7-16. Abdominal incisions.

of this scrubbing renders the operative site surgically clean but not sterile. The responsibility for doing the "prep" varies; the circulating nurse, the surgeon, or one of the assistants will do this skin preparation. The setups and solutions used will vary from hospital to hospital, but the basic procedure remains the same.

If the operative area is a flat surface, sterile towels may be used to localize this area. (Common abdominal incisional sites are shown in Fig. 7-16.) The scrubbing of the skin usually begins at the line of the proposed incision and proceeds outward to the periphery, or from "clean to dirty." This basic step is repeated, each time with a new gauze square or sponge. The sponge used to scrub should never go from the periphery back to the center of the operative site.

The site to be scrubbed often contains an area that may harbor bacteria not normally found on the skin. This could be a colostomy, draining sinus, ulcer, anus, or umbilicus. Care must be taken to assure that these bacteria are not spread out over the operative area. If possible, this area should be sealed off; if this is not possible, it should be scrubbed last. The sponge should be used once and discarded.

The purpose of draping is to provide a sterile field around the operative site. A minimal area of skin should be left exposed. Drapes may be of cotton muslin or synthetic disposable material. The synthetic materials have many advantages. They are soft, lint-free, lightweight, prepackaged, sterile, and ready for use. They should also be flame- and moisture-resistant. The light weight of these drapes prevents heat retention by the patient.

Towels or synthetic, adhering materials are used to drape the area immediately surrounding the operative site. When towels are used, the folded edge is placed toward the incisional site. Towels may be held in place with towel clips.

Draping sheets usually come in two sizes—half sheets and full sheets. They are used to cover the areas above and below the operative area or to drape for orthopedic procedures.

Fenestrated sheets are made with openings of varying sizes to both drape the patient and leave a particular site exposed. Examples are laparotomy (lap), kidney, thyroid, and chest sheets.

Perineal sheets (also fenestrated) are used to drape the patient who is in the lithotomy position. Leggings may be sewn to the sheet or be separate.

Whether linen or synthetic drapes are used, the same basic principles should be followed:

1. Drapes should be handled as little as possible.
2. Draping must never involve reaching over an unsterile area.
3. Draping sheets must not be allowed to fall below waist level because the area below the waist is always considered unsterile.
4. Drapes should be carried unfolded to the operative site. They must be held high enough to avoid touching unsterile sheets.
5. The incisional area is draped first, followed by draping to the periphery.
6. Once a drape is placed, it must not be moved. It should be discarded if it has not been placed correctly.
7. The gloved hand is protected with a cuff formed from the drape. The patient's skin is not touched.
8. Once a towel clip has been secured through a drape or to the patient's skin, it should be considered contaminated and discarded along with the drape if it is necessary to remove a drape during the procedure.
9. Whenever sterility is in doubt, the object is considered contaminated. "When in doubt, throw it out!"

INSTRUMENTATION

Instruments come in a variety of sizes and shapes based on their purpose. An instrument room may look very formidable to a new nurse in the operating room. However the nurse will find that they can be divided into groups *by use* such as *cutting, clamping, grasping, exposing,* and *suturing.* There is no standard nomenclature for instruments, and each manufacturer selects a name for his own design. An instrument may also be named after its originator (usually a surgeon).

Selection of instruments for an operative procedure depends on the size of the patient, anatomy involved, special technics, and preferences of the surgeon. One way to select instruments is to visualize the procedure

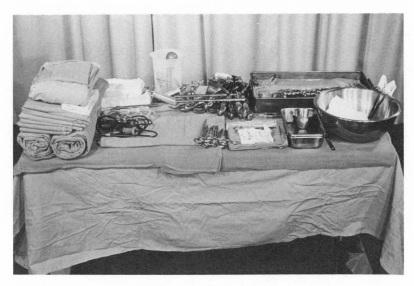

Fig. 7-17. Typical major procedure set-up.

step by step and select the appropriate instruments. Each instrument is designed for a specific use and should be used for that purpose only. Fig. 7-17 shows a variety of instruments included on a typical major table setup.

Cutting or *dissecting* instruments include scalpels, scissors, bone cutters, rongeurs, chisels, osteotomes, dermatomes, tonsillectomes, adenotomes, snares, saws, curettes, and vein strippers.

Clamping instruments include all hemostatic clamps, gallbladder forceps, stomach and intestinal clamps, blood vessel clamps, and other clamps designed for use on specific organs.

Grasping instruments include all tissue forceps, towel clamps, tenacula, bone holders, rib approximators, and stone forceps.

Exposing instruments include all retractors, dilators, specula, and endoscopy instruments.

Suturing instruments include needles, needle holders, wound clips, stapling devices, or any instrument used to hold a wound together.

Instrument usage

Each instrument has been designed for a particular purpose, and it should be used for that purpose only (for example, hemostats should not be used as pliers).

Most scalpels used today are actually knife handles with removable, disposable blades. These blades are prepackaged sterile in a variety of sizes and shapes ready for use.

Hemostats are designed to occlude blood vessels and come in a large variety of sizes and shapes. The jaws may be curved or straight and the serrations may be transverse or longitudinal. Special jaws that have fine-meshed, multiple rows of teeth arranged longitudinally instead of the usual serration have been made for occluding blood vessels. These fine-meshed teeth prevent leakage and minimize trauma to the vessel walls.

Holding instruments, tenacula, and tissue holding forceps are equipped with multiple fine teeth or with fine serrations. They are designed to hold tissue. Other holding instruments are towel clamps. They have sharp, curved jaws that penetrate tissue or drapes and are damaging to both.

Care of instruments

1. Instruments should be inspected before and after use. Damaged instruments should be set aside for repair or replacement. A damaged instrument could endanger a patient's life.
2. Instruments should have regular maintenance such as sharpening.
3. Instruments should be cleaned meticulously. Instrument washers and sonic cleaners are both good for cleaning. Instruments must not be exposed to corrosive chemicals.
4. Instruments should be clean and thoroughly dried before storing.
5. Instruments should not be oiled. Oil forms a film that prevents effective sterilization. It is also difficult to remove.
6. The edges of sharp instruments must be protected. Dropping or jamming against other instruments is to be avoided.
7. Lensed instruments require special care. Autoclaving will damage them, and the solvent in some chemical disinfectants will dissolve the cement holding the lens. Metal and plastic parts must be protected. These instruments are introduced into body cavities and sharp edges can cause tissue damage.
8. All parts of instruments (particularly self-retaining retractors) must be accounted for before, during, and after the procedure. Some instruments have screws, nuts, and other small pieces that could become dislodged and left in a patient.

SUTURES AND NEEDLES

Sutures serve two purposes: (1) to tie off vessels in order to control bleeding, and (2) to hold tissues together until they heal. Suture materials are either absorbable or nonabsorbable in body tissues.

Absorbable sutures, most of which are commonly called "catgut," are sutures that are broken down and dissolved by enzymes produced by the body. "Catgut" is a misnomer, since this material is made from submucosa of sheep intestine or serosa of beef intestine. Synthetic absorbable sutures have recently become available.

A tanning or chromicizing process delays the absorption rate of *chromic* catgut. *Plain* catgut is untreated and is absorbed more rapidly than the treated suture.

Nonabsorbable suture is not dissolved by enzymes. This suture remains encapsulated in tissue or is removed when used as a skin closure. Nonabsorbable sutures are made of metal, organic material, or synthetics. An easy way to remember the types of sutures is that absorbable suture is temporary and nonabsorbable suture is permanent.

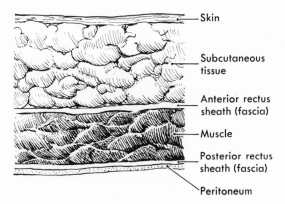

Fig. 7-18. Layers of abdominal wall tissue to be sutured following abdominal surgery.

Sizes of sutures range from 10-0 to 4; 10-0 is the smallest in diameter. The size used will depend on the kind of tissue and the purpose of the suture. The very fine suture is used in eye, vascular, or plastic surgery, whereas the very heavy suture is used for retention purposes. Fig. 7-18 illustrates the layers of abdominal wall tissue. Each of these layers might require a different type and size of suture material. The fascia surrounding muscles, rather than the muscle tissue itself, is usually sutured.

Needles are selected according to the tissue and vessels to be sutured, the location, and accessibility. Needle points are taper (noncutting) or cutting. Variations of the cutting point include triangular, trocar, or spear. The basic shapes are straight, half-curved, half-circle and three-eights circle. Sizes of needles are utterly confusing. The number may refer to either the distance between the eye of the needle and point or the length of the steel before the needle is made.

Before needles are placed in instrument sets, they should be checked to be sure that the points are sharp and the eyes are intact. Use of disposable needles is becoming increasingly popular today.

Some surgeons prefer swaged-on needles. Swaged-on needles cause less trauma than threaded needles because only one width of the suture passes through the tissue. In addition, the needle is used only once and, therefore, is always sharp. Nursing time is saved since the needle-suture combination is ready for use from the package.

Terminology

continuous suture single suture used to join two wound edges and tied at each end
interrupted suture single sutures placed and tied separately
ligature or **tie** suture material used to close off ends of severed blood vessels; may be single strands or continuous from a reel
stick tie or **suture ligature** suture material on a needle used to ligate a blood vessel
retention suture heavy nonabsorbable suture used to reinforce a wound where unusual stress on the suture line is anticipated
swaged-on or **atraumatic suture** suture attached to an eyeless needle during the manu-

facturing process; advantages are lessened tissue trauma, sharp needles, and no unthreading of suture

HEMOSTASIS

The loss of blood may mean the loss of life. In ancient times hemorrhage was controlled by pouring boiling oil into a wound or searing it with hot irons. This caused indescribable suffering, infection, and permanent disability, along with a high mortality rate. Today, of course, the methods are quite refined in comparison.

It is generally thought that clotting takes place by an enzyme reaction. Injured tissues release thromboplastin, and prothrombin is normally present in blood. Prothrombin, thromboplastin, and calcium ions in the blood form thrombin. Within a short time thrombin combines with fibrinogen, a blood protein, to form fibrin. Fibrin forms the basic structure of a clot.

Even though the ligature was known by Hippocrates, he used and recommended cautery (hot irons) because he knew infection did not occur as often when cautery was used. The use of ligatures was then temporarily forgotten until the second century when Galen began using them again. After trying all other methods, Ambrose Pare, in the sixteenth century, used ligatures to stop bleeding after amputations.

Many of our present methods of hemostasis are based on the same principles as those used by the ancient surgeons. Today, however, the methods of hemostasis cause a minimum of trauma to tissue and do not cause infection.

Methods of hemostasis

Pressure. Pressure is one of the quickest, easiest, and most effective methods of stopping bleeding, whether the bleeding area is small or quite extensive. Pressure is used on the bleeding point, either manually or by firm dressings and bandages. It is believed that pressure delays hemorrhage until clotting occurs.

Hemostat (*hemo*, blood; *stat*, stop). Hemostats come in a variety of sizes and shapes, but they all serve the purpose of clamping off a bleeding vessel.

Electrocoagulation. Electrocoagulation is the present-day method of searing small blood vessels to control bleeding. A commonly used unit is the Bovie unit. The Bovie is a machine used to cut tissue and to coagulate bleeding points by high frequency current. This current passes through the patient's body between two electrodes.

Certain precautions must be observed when using a cautery unit: (1) the patient must be properly grounded; (2) the unit cannot be used when certain explosive anesthetic agents are being used; (3) alcohol or flammable liquids must not be used near a cautery; (4) only the necessary amount of current is to be employed; (5) when cautery is used in the bladder, water or normal saline solutions cannot be used, since these solutions act as conductors and disperse the current.

Ligatures. Ligatures are suture materials used to tie around vessels that have been clamped by hemostats.

Bone wax. Bone wax is composed mainly of beeswax. It is used to seal bleeders in bone.

Heat. Hot packs may be used occasionally to control capillary bleeding in extensive procedures such as a radical mastectomy.

Oxidized cellulose (Oxycel, Surgicel). This absorbable hemostatic agent is made of gauze or cotton. It is placed over a bleeding area and is usually not removed. It absorbs blood, swells, and becomes sticky and jelly-like, forming coagulum. The hemostatic action results from the coagulum and pressure exerted by the swelling of the cellulose.

Thrombin. Thrombin is an extracted fraction of beef blood. It accelerates coagulation of blood and may be used as a powder or mixed into a solution.

Gelatin sponge. This absorbable sponge is made from specially cured and sterilized gelatin. The sponge is placed on an area of capillary bleeding and fibrin is formed. The sponge swells, forming a sizable clot. Gelatin sponge comes in a variety of forms (sponge, powder, or film) and sizes. It can be cut without crumbling.

Styptic. Styptic is a chemical that causes constriction or contraction of blood vessels. Two examples are epinephrine, which is used alone or with local anesthetics, and tannic acid powder, which is used on mucous membranes.

Clips. Clips may be used to occlude the lumen of a blood vessel to stop bleeding.

Vitamin K. This essential vitamin may be administered preoperatively and postoperatively to supplement body stores needed in coagulation of blood and tissue repair.

DOCUMENTATION OF NURSING CARE

Nursing care of the patient in the operating room is not complete without documentation of that care. Not only does this aid continuity of care, but it also helps operating room nurses identify nursing actions that contribute to safety and comfort for the patient.

Operating room nursing care can be recorded in the patient's chart as part of the ongoing record. In some hospitals special operating room record forms are used. Whatever the format, documented patient information should include: time of arrival in operating room, level of consciousness, behavioral description of emotional state, intravenous site (including needle/cannula) and intravenous solutions, arm positions on armboard, positioning and devices used, skin condition pre- and postoperatively, site of placement of electrocautery ground pads and monitor electrodes, area prepped and solution used, surgical procedure performed, cultures and specimens, irrigating solutions, medications, blood given, drains and catheters, unusual happenings or complications, dressings, and time and method of transfer to recovery area.[1]

REFERENCE

1. Mehaffy, N. L.: Assessment and communication for continuity of care for the surgical patient, Nurs. Clin. North Am. 10(4):630-632, Dec. 1975.

SUGGESTED READINGS

Ahlstrom, G., and Ahlstrom, H.: Hospital's instrument problems—and some suggestions for relief, AORN J. 15:77-87, Jan. 1972.

Ballinger, W. F., Treybal, J. C., and Vose, A. B.: Alexander's care of the patient in surgery, ed. 5, St. Louis, 1972, The C. V. Mosby Co.

Bergerson, B. S.: Pharmacology in nursing, ed. 13, St. Louis, 1976, The C. V. Mosby Co.

Birch, A. A., and Tolmie, J. D., editors: Anesthesia for the uninterested, Baltimore, 1976, University Park Press.

Brooks, S. M.: Fundamentals of operating room nursing, St. Louis, 1975, The C. V. Mosby Co.

Care and handling of surgical instruments, Randolph, Mass., 1969, Codman & Shurtleff, Inc.

Carey, J., and Smith, R. M.: Needles, past, present and future, AORN J. 16:209-216, Oct. 1972.

Cohen, E. Cleaner air for the OR, Mod. Health Care, pp. 82-83, Nov. 1974.

Cohen, E.: Occupational disease among operating room personnel: A national study, Anesthesiology 41:321-340, Oct. 1974.

DeLappe, A.: Shhh! Sleeping patients are listening, AORN J. 19:1334-1348, June 1974.

Federal standards on waste anesthetic gases being prepared, AORN J. 20:950-951, Dec. 1974.

Genereux, T. B.: Positioning OR patients in the operating room, Am. J. Nurs. 59:1572-1574, Nov. 1959.

Gruendemann, B. J.: Social structure of hospital operating rooms, AORN J. 11:43-48, May 1970.

Lach, J.: OR Nursing: Preoperative care and draping technique, Chicago, 1974, Kendall Co.

MacClelland, D. C.: Are current skin preparations valid? AORN J. 21:55-60, Jan. 1975.

Minckley, B.: Physiological hazards of position changes in the anesthetized patient, Am. J. Nurs. 69:2606-2611, Dec. 1969.

Nursing care of the patient in the O.R., Somerville, New Jersey, 1972, Ethicon, Inc.

Robertson, P. A.: Respiratory care in local anesthesia, AORN J. 21:797-805, April 1975.

Robinchon, P.: The challenge of crisis theory for nursing, Nurs. Outlook 15:28-32, July 1967.

Rosenberg, H., Guest, D., and Etsten, B.: Forane—Experience with the newest inhalation agent, Anesthesiology Rev., Oct. 1974.

Scott, W. E.: Anesthesia for open heart surgery, AORN J. 20:1060-1068, Dec. 1974.

Stubbs, D. H.: Anesthesiology—What nurses should know about it, AORN J. 4:75-81, July-Aug. 1966.

Waste anesthetic gas suspect as OR health hazard, AORN J. 20:754-756, Nov. 1974.

CHAPTER 8

IMMEDIATE POSTANESTHESIA CARE

One of the most critical times for a patient can be the time from the completion of surgery to his admission to the recovery, or postanesthesia, room. Moving the patient from the operating room table to the recovery bed can be hazardous. A minimum of four people is needed to move the patient and keep his body in proper alignment during the transfer. Moving a patient rapidly can be dangerous; care must be taken to see that the patient does not slip between the table and the bed or have a leg or arm caught or scraped. Patient rollers are available and especially helpful when moving a heavy patient. Operating room personnel should also use good body mechanics to prevent injury to themselves.

Busy personnel sometimes lose interest in the patient after he is moved from the operating room table to the recovery bed. The surgeon leaves to write his orders and postoperative note; the anesthesiologist is busy completing his records; and the nursing personnel may be busy cleaning the room in preparation for the next surgery. This is a time when hypotension and cardiac arrest can occur in the patient. Change in position may cause respiratory obstruction or stimulate vomiting. Therefore, observation of the patient and constant attendance are necessary at this crucial time.

Postanesthesia recovery rooms have played and will continue to play a most important role in reducing mortality rates of the immediate postoperative period. The postanesthesia room provides an area where patients emerging from anesthesia (general, regional, or local) can be observed closely until they have regained consciousness and/or their condition stabilizes. This may be an hour or less; in some hospitals, patients are kept overnight.

This special area or room should be located immediately adjacent to the operating room so that the patient is transported a minimal distance. In addition, surgeons and anesthesiologists are near and can be summoned quickly should emergencies arise. It is important that surgeons and operating room personnel have easy access to the recovery room. Also, a

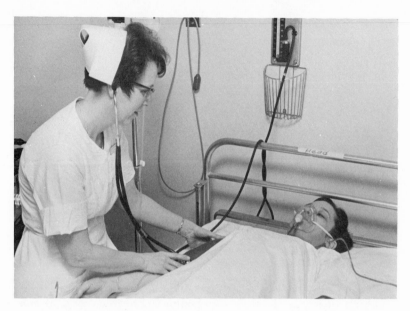

Fig. 8-1. Patient being admitted to the postanesthesia unit.

space within the room should be available for patients who must be isolated.

As soon as the patient is admitted to the postanesthesia, or recovery, room, the nurse immediately ascertains his condition (Fig. 8-1). A report is obtained from the anesthesiologist. This report includes type and extent of the operation, types of anesthetic agents and drugs used, and any complications that might have occurred in surgery. It is most important that the nurse know what drugs were administered, because smaller doses of narcotics are necessary with some drugs, whereas the use of other drugs necessitates special nursing care. Each nurse should know the precautions that must be taken.

The operating room nurse should also be present when the patient is admitted to the recovery room to give a nursing report to the recovery room nurse. They may review the care plan together and discuss findings and highlights of the surgery.

As mentioned in Chapter 7, hearing is the last sense to be abolished as the patient is anesthetized. The sense of hearing is also one of the first to be restored as the patient recovers from anesthesia. Personnel must always be aware of their conversations, especially when they involve findings of surgery or aspects of patient care. Even though a patient appears to be sleeping, he may later astound the nurse with his recollections of the recovery room. Therefore, any discussions about the patient should take place in an area away from his bed.

One of the most important attributes of the expert recovery room nurse is the power of astute observation. This means knowing when the patient is reacting and recovering normally from anesthesia and being alert to *every change* in the patient's condition. The recovery room nurse must be able to think and act quickly and in a perceptive and professional manner. The nurse is always prepared for emergencies and has equipment ready and in working condition.

Immediately upon admission to the recovery room, the nurse should determine the patient's condition by noting the following:

1. *Respirations.* Check rate, rhythm, and depth. Determine if the patient has an adequate airway and if respiratory exchange is satisfactory. (Placing the hand above the patient's nose and mouth to feel for exhaled air is one simple way of grossly determining the air exchange.) Give oxygen according to patient's needs and the physician's orders. To determine the need for oxygen, check the color of the skin, lips, and nail beds; note pulse rate and compare with the basal reading obtained preoperatively.

If the airway is inadequate:

a. Hyperextend the patient's head and bring chin forward.

b. Turn the patient to one side to avoid aspiration of secretions.

c. Insert nasopharyngeal or oropharyngeal airway.

d. Suction mucus and secretions that pool in naso- or oropharynx.

e. Encourage the patient to cough and deep breathe if he is able.

2. *Pulse.* Check rate, quality, and regularity of rhythm. If arrhythmia is present, record and notify surgeon. It is important to compare the pulse rate with the basal rate obtained before surgery. Cardiac monitors may be used.

3. *Blood pressure.* If blood pressure is abnormally high or low, consult the surgery record to note readings during the operation. If there is a wide discrepancy, it should be reported immediately. The nurse must also check the operative area and entire dressing for bleeding and excessive drainage.

4. *Skin.* Check color and condition (pale, pink, flushed, cyanotic, warm, dry, hot, moist).

5. *Intravenous fluids.* Check to see if fluids are infusing satisfactorily and at the rate ordered. Make notation of the kind of fluids and amount given. If blood is infusing, watch for signs and symptoms of a transfusion reaction (nausea, urticaria, increase in pulse rate or respirations, hypertension, apprehension or fever); if noted, stop blood infusion and call the surgeon.

6. *Drainage tubes.* Check for patency. Urethral, ureteral, and suprapubic catheters should be connected to proper drainage or irrigation if ordered. Nasogastric tubes should be connected to drainage or suction. Suction catheters should be connected to suction of the recommended negative pressure. Thoracotomy tubes (see number 9 below) will be attached to underwater drainage before the patient leaves the operating room. It is most important that the chest drainage bottle is never lifted

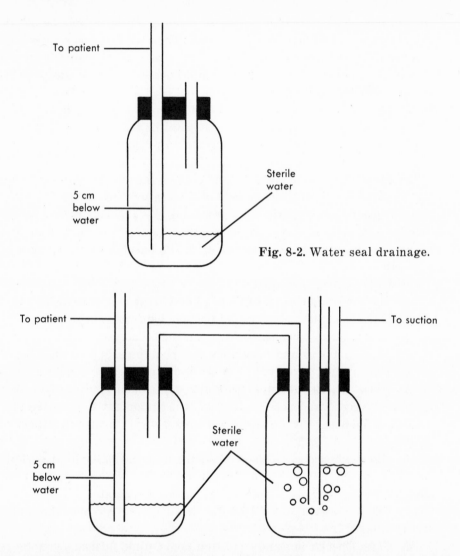

Fig. 8-2. Water seal drainage.

Fig. 8-3. Water seal suction. The first bottle provides a water seal and collects drainage. The second bottle provides suction control. Depth of tube under water will determine negative pressure.

to or above the chest level. This would cause water in the bottles to be sucked into the chest cavity, causing contamination and collapse of the lung with very serious consequences. Amount, color, and consistency of all drainage should be noted and charted.

7. *Position.* The optimal position is one that permits drainage of respiratory and gastric secretions and prevents respiratory obstruction. The patient should be in the lateral position with the head slightly down. The tongue will be forward in the mouth to ensure an adequate airway. Secretions can drain outside of the mouth or pool in the side of the mouth

where they can be suctioned out. A steep head-down position will cause the abdominal contents to fall against the diaphragm and may limit the depth of respirations. A patient in the supine position must be watched closely. The pharyngeal muscles are relaxed and the tongue may occlude the airway. Regurgitated liquids pool in the pharynx and may be aspirated by the patient as long as the swallowing reflex is absent.

8. *Consciousness.* The state of consciousness and orientation of the patient must be noted, especially as the patient begins to recover from the anesthesia.

9. *Chest drainage.* Patients arriving in the postanesthesia room after a thoracotomy will probably have chest tubes attached to water seal drainage. The two basic types of water seal drainage are gravity and suction drainage (Figs. 8-2 and 8-3). If suction drainage is used, a Gomco type of electric suction or suction regulator for the wall suction will be necessary.

The purpose of chest drainage is to (1) remove air and drainage of blood from the intrapleural space, (2) expand the lung on the operative side, and (3) restore subatmospheric pressure in the thoracic cavity. One or two chest tubes are usually used. They are positioned anterior and posterior to the axillary line in the eighth or ninth intercostal spaces. A third tube may be necessary if alveolar leakage is excessive. It is placed in the second interspace anteriorly. A separate drainage setup is needed for each chest tube.

A one, two, or three bottle drainage system may be used. The one bottle system works by gravity. The tip of the water seal chest tube must be kept under water. It is important that this bottle be kept 60 to 90 cm. below patient's chest. If not, the water in the bottle could be sucked into the chest cavity.

The two bottle system is used when a persistent air leak cannot be controlled by drainage alone and a water seal suction is necessary. The extra bottle acts as a suction regulator, maintaining the intensity of suction to minus 10 to 20 cm. of water. Direct suction would pull lung tissue against the holes of the chest tube, thereby occluding it.

Important nursing considerations are:

1. All equipment must be sterile and sterility maintained.
2. The system must be airtight.
3. The bottles must be kept below the patient's chest.
4. Clamps for the tubes should always be with the patient, at the bedside.

POSSIBLE COMPLICATIONS AND POSTOPERATIVE CONDITIONS
Cardiovascular complications

Hypotension is the most common postoperative complication. It is usually caused by decreased circulating blood volume. Patients will vary in their ability to tolerate hypovolemia. Chronically ill or debilitated patients may already have a decreased blood volume and may not tolerate even a small loss of blood. Methods to measure blood loss are still not reliable, and estimations of blood loss are frequently inaccurate.

Many drugs used as anesthetics (both general and local) decrease peripheral vascular resistance and cause the blood to pool peripherally. This predisposes to hypotension.

Sudden changes in position may shift the blood volume away from the heart, leading to cardiovascular collapse. Tight abdominal dressings or increased intrathoracic pressure produced by positive-pressure respiration may cause mechanical interference with venous flow and hypotension.

Other less common causes of hypotension are pulmonary embolism, transfusion reactions, and myocardial infarction, which may occur during or just after an operation.

Cardiac arrest

Cardiopulmonary arrest is the sudden and unexpected cessation of respirations and functional circulation. The causes of cardiac arrest are many. Among them are cardiogenic shock, electric shock, idiosyncratic response to anesthetic agents, drug sensitivity, central nervous system trauma, drug overdose, or anything that will cause hypercarbia or anoxia; ventricular fibrillation or standstill; or inadequate circulating blood volume. Two major causes of cardiac arrest in the operating room are hypovolemic shock and respiratory obstruction from laryngospasm or from aspiration of obstructing material such as vomitus or blood.

Prevention of this complication is the responsibility of everyone assisting in the operating room. This requires that nursing personnel use care in positioning, moving, and transporting patients. There must be a well-trained postanesthesia room staff that has adequate equipment and knows how to use that equipment. Preoperative evaluation and preparation of patients and the selection of preoperative medications and appropriate anesthesia are the responsibility of the medical staff.

Early signs of cardiac arrest are seldom clearly defined. Signs and symptoms include loss of consciousness, disorientation, anxiety, dyspnea, cyanosis, pallor, gasping breaths, laryngeal stricture, hypotension, weak and irregular pulse, and dilated pupils. Dilation of the pupils begins 45 seconds after circulation ceases and is complete within 2 minutes.

If the patient has no pulses, respiration, or blood pressure and has dilated pupils, he is in cardiopulmonary arrest. The success of treatment depends on rapid action. The nurse must know what to do, know how to do it, and do it without delay.

The ABC's of resuscitation are:

Airway: This is the most important step of successful resuscitation. Tilt the head backward and displace the jaw forward.

Breathing: Positive pressure ventilation must be started immediately, using mouth-to-mouth or mouth-to-nose resuscitation, breathing bags, or respirators.

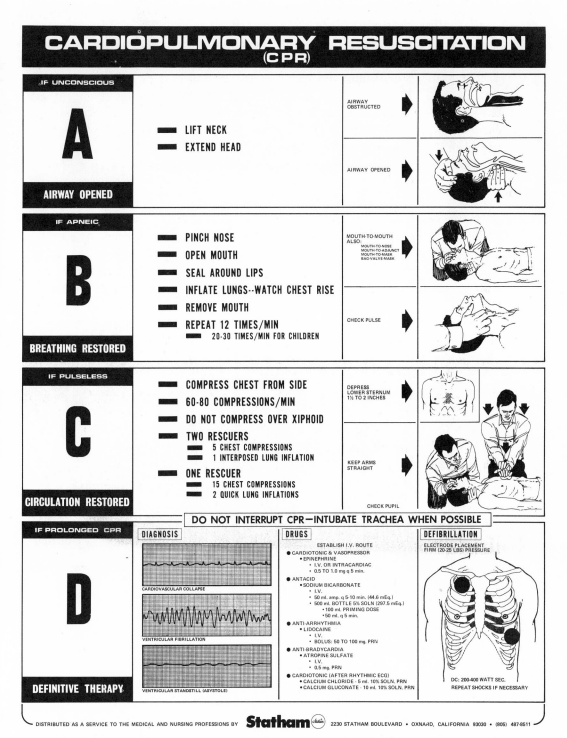

Fig. 8-4. Cardiopulmonary resuscitation. (Reproduced with permission from Statham Instruments, Inc., Oxnard, California.)

Circulation: External cardiac massage must be started immediately. Open cardiac massage is rarely used outside the operating room.

Definitive therapy should be initiated as soon as possible. Cardiac monitoring equipment is used. Intravenous fluids should be started and an endotracheal tube inserted to ensure an adequate supply of oxygen and exchange of gases. Defibrillation or cardioversion is done when indicated. Calcium chloride, 10%, or epinephrine, 1:10,000, may be given intracardially. The following drugs may be given intravenously: sodium bicarbonate, lidocaine, isoproterenol (Isuprel), levarterenol (Levophed), atropine sulfate, calcium chloride, or calcium gluconate.

The steps in cardiopulmonary resuscitation are shown in Fig. 8-4.

Shock

Shock is a condition of inadequate tissue perfusion. Examples of causes include blood loss or loss of body fluids following severe diarrhea or vomiting.

Shock can be classified into six basic categories: (1) hypovolemic, (2) neurogenic, (3) traumatic, (4) septic, (5) anaphylactic, and (6) cardiogenic.

Hypovolemic shock may be the result of hemorrhage caused by trauma or gastrointestinal bleeding. Loss of plasma volume is the result of severe diarrhea, vomiting, or burns. The venous return decreases and causes the cardiac output to decrease, lowering tissue perfusion.

Neurogenic shock is caused by brain damage, deep anesthesia, or overdoses of narcotics that depress the vasomotor centers in the medulla, causing the loss of neurogenic tone to vessels. This produces vasodilatation, which reduces blood pressure and circulating blood volume.

Traumatic shock is caused by contusion of body tissues, which damages capillaries, causing plasma leakage into tissues, thus reducing plasma volume. Pain caused by trauma may inhibit the vasomotor center, thereby producing vasodilatation.

Septic shock is caused by bacterial infection that produces vasodilatation, blood stasis, and cardiac depression.

Anaphylactic shock is produced by antigen-antibody reactions that damage tissue and most cells. This releases toxic substances such as histamine, which is a potent vasodilator.

Cardiogenic shock is caused by damage to the heart muscle because of myocardial infarct or heart attack. This damage weakens the pumping action, which decreases cardiac output.

Clinical signs for all types of shock are essentially the same: diminished or absent brachial arterial pressure; diminished or absent brachial and radial pulses; cool, clammy extremities and peripheral cyanosis; decreased urine output; and alterations in mental state varying from agitation to apathy and coma. Rapid respirations and tachycardia may be present except in the elderly. In hypertensive patients the systolic pressure may be in the normal range but would be low for the patient's normal needs.

Treatment will vary according to the cause of shock. In hypovolemic shock, fluid replacement of lost volume with blood, plasma, plasma expanders, or low molecular weight dextrans is essential. The amount of fluid administered should be governed by the increase in blood pressure. Excessive amounts of fluids will cause pulmonary edema.

Treatment of other types of shock will vary according to the underlying cause. All patients in shock should be monitored on the electrocardiogram, and given oxygen and intravenous fluids. Elevating the foot of the bed may help.

Cardiac arrhythmias

Many patients are saved because an alert nurse recognized and initiated treatment of cardiac arrhythmias (Table 4). This can be especially important in the operating room and recovery room since some anesthetic drugs and gases may cause arrhythmias. Early diagnosis and treatment are extremely important, but equally important is knowing what *not* to do; for example, cardioversion for some patients taking digitalis may cause lethal arrhythmias.

Pulmonary complications

Pulmonary complications are frequent and probably the most serious of all complications. Narcotics, many sedatives, and most of the commonly used inhalation anesthetics depress respirations. During the operation a patient's respirations are frequently supported by the anesthesiologist, either manually or by mechanical respirators. At the close of the procedure these methods are stopped and the patient is expected to control his own respirations.

To provide surgical relaxation, neuromuscular blocking agents such as succinylcholine or curare may be used. These may cause some degree of respiratory difficulty during the postoperative period. High spinals or epidural anesthesia may also cause respiratory paralysis. The action of curare-type drugs can be reversed with neostigmine or edrophonium chloride (Tensilon), but the only treatment for the other types of respiratory paralysis is to support respirations artifically until adequate respiration returns.

Another very important cause of postoperative respiratory insufficiency is obstruction of the airway. The most frequent obstruction is pharyngeal or laryngeal. This can be corrected by tilting the head and supporting the jaw to pull the tongue away from the posterior pharynx, or an oral or nasal airway can be inserted. Another cause is aspiration of gastric secretions, mucus, blood, teeth, artificial bridges, or even chewing gum. Some limitation of respiratory excursion may be caused by pain. This will vary depending on the surgical procedure. The pattern of respirations may

Table 4. Cardiac arrhythmias

	Rate/rhythm	ECG changes	Interpretations	Treatment
Sinus arrhythmia	Slower than normal Irregular	P wave: normal PR interval: normal QRS complex: normal	Usually seen in children Related to respiratory cycle Heart rate increases with inspiration; decreases with expiration	None
Sinus tachycardia	110 to 180/minute Children may exceed 200 Slightly irregular	P wave: normal; may be difficult to identify	Common causes—anxiety, fever, and shock Increases cardiac output, which may cause pulmonary embolism, congestive heart failure	Treat underlying cause No cardiac drugs
Sinus bradycardia	Below 60/minute Usually irregular	P wave: normal PR: within upper limits of normal QRS: normal	Normal in well trained athletes Seen in patients on morphine, digitalis, or pressor amines Watch for congestive heart failure, ventricular irritability, or cardiac arrest	Atropine 0.5 to 1 mg. IV Isoproterenol Transvenous pacing
Sinus arrest	Slower than normal Irregular	P wave: absent PR: absent QRS: absent	Caused by drugs (e.g., quinidine, procaine amide, digitalis) Increased vagal tone	Discontinue drugs Begin transvenous pacing
Paroxysmal atrial tachycardia (PAT)	150 to 250/minute Regular	P wave: abnormal, often difficult to identify PR: prolonged QRS: normal	Seen in young adults; patients complain of pounding in chest or breathlessness May cause myocardial ischemia or congestive heart failure	Stimulation of vagal nerve by massaging right carotid sinus or gag patient Fast acting digitalis preparation Cardioversion may be necessary

Arrhythmia	Rate/Rhythm	ECG	Significance	Treatment
Atrial flutter	250 to 350/minute Regular	P wave: absent; replaced by flutter waves PR: variable QRS: normal or aberrant	Usually occurs in arteriosclerotic or rheumatic patient Causes congestive heart failure, myocardial ischemia	Digitalis, quinidine, or cardioversion Digitalis slows pulse rate by blocking AV node If patient is on digitalis, cardioversion may cause lethal arrhythmia
Atrial fibrillation	300 to 500/minute Atrial rate usually faster than ventricular rate Irregular	P wave: irregular PR: absent QRS: normal or aberrant	Myocardial ischemia, congestive heart failure	Digitalis, propranolol, cardioversion
Ventricular tachycardia	100 to 200/minute Usually regular	P wave: present; may be difficult to identify PR: no fixed relationship QRS: abnormal; wide	May be caused by digitalis or myocardial depressant drugs, electrolyte imbalance, myocardial ischemia, or infarction Excessive fluids may cause congestive failure	Lidocaine—bolus or IV drip Cardioversion may be necessary
Ventricular fibrillation	Rapid; variable atrial; absent ventricular Irregular	P wave: absent PR: absent QRS: abnormal, asymmetric	Caused by acute myocardial infarction Patient has no pulse Death will result in minutes if arrhythmia is not terminated immediately	Defibrillation Lidocaine Treatment must be instituted immediately

change after upper abdominal or thoracic procedures. The respiratory pattern will be rapid and shallow, and the chest will be held in the expiratory position.

Some degree of microatelectasis always occurs as a result of inhaling anesthetic egents. This may become more serious if pneumothorax also occurs. Pneumothorax is a rare but serious emergency whereas atelectasis is a common aftermath of general anesthesia. Coughing and deep breathing, as discussed in Chapter 6, are of tremendous value to the patient if he remembers to do this as he was taught during the preoperative visit. The coughing and deep breathing exercises are specifically intended to inflate the areas of atelectasis in the lungs so that oxygenation improves.

Postoperative pain

Pain is the least understood and probably the most serious postoperative complication from the patient's viewpoint. Causes of pain are many and varied. The patient's psychologic makeup, his family relationships, the expected results of the surgery, and the type of incision and amount of organ manipulation all have much to do with the amount of pain a patient experiences. The removal of a painful, acutely inflamed appendix is a relief, but the disfiguring results of some operations for cancer will tend to cause the patient to feel more pain. Patients who have been told what to expect usually have less pain than those who have not been informed. Narcotics are usually used for relief of pain, but because they are respiratory depressants, the dosage should be reduced while the patient is still in the immediate postoperative period.

Increased intracranial pressure

Increased intracranial pressure is a frequent complication following craniotomies. Evaluation of the neurologic status is an important aspect of postoperative care following a craniotomy. Changes in neurologic signs will usually precede changes in vital signs.

Frequent monitoring of vital signs is important. These should be checked every 15 to 30 minutes for the first 3 to 4 hours postoperatively, then every hour if the patient's condition seems to be stabilizing. Cardinal signs of increased intracranial pressure are slow pulse, hypertension, and irregular, slow respirations.

Evaluation of the patient's neurologic status (in any operation) may indicate the presence of a complication. The long-lasting effects of a general anesthetic may confuse the diagnosis. Signs to watch for are continued vomiting or retching, abnormal respirations, unstable blood pressure, rapid pulse, deterioration in state of consciousness, hemiparesis, and dilated, fixed pupils.

A patient who has lapsed into unconsciousness may develop an obstructed airway, and cerebral hypoxia will result. Hypoxia will then cause further deterioration and aggravate cerebral edema.

SUMMARY

Preoperative visit records and nursing care guides can be very helpful for operating room and postanesthesia room personnel. Understanding a patient's emotional needs and knowing his physical disabilities will make nursing care much easier and more patient centered. The patient who has been instructed preoperatively will know for example, why he must deep breathe, that he may have intravenous fluids, what drains or tubes may be required, and that he may receive medications for discomfort and pain if needed.

The nurse in the postanesthesia unit plays a vital role in providing a smooth, safe postoperative course for the patient.

SUGGESTED READINGS

Butler, H.: How to read an ECG, Oradell, N.J., 1973, Medical Economics Co.

Chow, R. K.: Cardiosurgical nursing care, New York, 1976, Springer Publishing Co., Inc.

Civetta, J. M.: Recovery room: Past, present and future, AORN J. 21:806-811, April 1975.

Conover, M. H.: Cardiac arrhythmias: Exercises in pattern interpretation, St. Louis, 1974, The C. V. Mosby Co.

Dietzman, R., and others: Shock, J. Am. Coll. Emerg. Physicians, Mar.-April 1973.

Duban, D.: Rapid interpretation EKGs, 1970, Cover Publishing Co.

Fay, M. R.: Nursing process in the recovery room, AORN J. 24:1069-1075, Dec. 1976.

Harvey, A., and others: The principles and practice of medicine, New York, 1972, Appleton-Century-Crofts, pp. 456-461, 1518-1527.

Heimlich, H.: Understanding chest drainage by understanding breathing, Health Care 1:3-8, Oct. 1970.

Holley, H. S.: Anesthesia, Methods to recovery, AORN J. 21:822-835, April 1975.

Hurst, J. W., and Myerburg, R. J.: Electrocardiography, New York, 1968, McGraw-Hill, Inc.

Kroner, J. A.: OR/PAR cooperation for better patient care, AORN J. 23:181-182, Feb. 1976.

LeMaitre, G., and Finnegan, J.: The patient in surgery—A guide for nurses, ed. 2, Philadelphia, 1975, W. B. Saunders, Co., pp. 407-412.

Paradis, C. P.: Nursing in the recovery room, AORN J. 18:1117-1126, Dec. 1973.

Smith, B. J.: After anesthesia, Nursing '74 4:28-32, Dec. 1974.

Thorp, G.: Shock—The overall mechanism, Am. J. Nurs. 74:489-520, Dec. 1974.

Van Meter, M.: Chest tubes—Basic techniques for better care, Nursing '74 4:48-55, Dec. 1974.

CHAPTER 9

POSTOPERATIVE NURSING FOLLOW-UP

Total nursing care of the surgical patient involves three phases: preoperative, surgical, and postoperative care. By becoming involved in the preoperative and surgical phase of the patient's care the operating room nurse is committed to follow through into the postoperative phase. The nurse must do this in order to evaluate the effectiveness of the preoperative visit and also to reinforce the preoperative instructions.

Postoperative visits should be made until the nurse is satisfied that the patient is making satisfactory recovery or is making optimal adjustment to the level of recovery that can be expected according to the prognosis of his illness.

Postoperative visits will vary from patient to patient. For those undergoing a simple, uncomplicated procedure, the operating room nurse may find that one postoperative visit is sufficient. For those patients who have had complicated, extensive surgery, such as the transplant of an organ or a radical procedure for malignancy, a daily visit may be vitally necessary to see that the patient receives the benefits of good nursing care.

The postoperative visit by the operating room nurse does not take the place of any care given by the unit personnel. The operating room nurse complements this care. Because of her unique knowledge, the operating room nurse may act as a consultant. Together, the operating room nurse and the head nurse on the unit can plan the most effective care for the patient—each nurse has special knowledge to contribute to the care plan.

Each patient must be evaluated as an individual. The nurse must assess, plan, and implement a nursing care plan on a daily basis. No set or standard plan of action will suffice to meet the needs of all patients. As the nurse becomes increasingly familiar with various individual personalities, she will come to recognize that each person reacts to the surgical experience in a different way. The nurse will learn to recognize the underlying factors that determine the patient's behavioral response to his illness.

WHY THE OPERATING ROOM NURSE MAKES
POSTOPERATIVE VISITS

The operating room nurse is familiar with the patient and has developed a unique rapport with him during the preoperative visit. During this visit the nurse established herself in the patient's mind as one who is "in the know" by explaining what was going to happen to him before surgery. The nurse also promised to see the patient after surgery, and he will be looking forward to the visit. Patient expectations at this time will vary. Some will be well informed concerning their surgery and expected prognosis. Others will be minimally informed about their condition. When making a postoperative visit, the nurse should keep in mind the possibility of a patient who asks, "Nurse, what did they do to me in the operating room?" She may well wonder, "What do I do now?"

Patients have the right to know about their health status and, if patients want to ask questions, the nurse should be prepared to give answers. It is preferable to have the patient's physician provide this type of information, and usually this is the case. But occasionally the nurse will find herself committed to the role of informant. How much she tells the patient in response to his questions concerning his surgery will be based on an assessment of the patient's condition and his ability to comprehend the explanation and still be able to handle the situation created by his knowing. Nurses faced with this situation, although keeping in mind the old adage, "Discretion is the better part of valor," should not draw back from the patient's questions. Neither should they rush in with answers until the situation has been explored thoroughly. Casual questioning may reveal that the physician has already given the patient as much information as his judgment indicated the patient could handle. If this has not been the case, then the nurse is committed to proceed according to her judgment.

Aside from the rapport the operating room nurse has established with the patient, there is another factor in favor of having the operating room nurse visit patients postoperatively. Operating room nursing is this nurse's specialty, and no other nurse in the hospital is as knowledgeable about the various surgical procedures and what they involve. The nurse knows where the drains, catheters, or other tubes are located in the patient's body. She understands why he might be experiencing certain types of discomfort. The nurse can help him verbalize his anxieties and, with her specific knowledge, can relieve many of these anxieties with a simple explanation.

Each patient responds differently following surgery; some patients have very little discomfort. Others exhibit mild to severe complications caused by pain, infection, or poor healing processes. Still other complications involve psychologic manifestations that require the combined skill of every member of the medical and nursing staff in order to return the patient to optimal psychologic and physiologic health.

Hosp. no. 775-1334 Age 50 Physicians Wright / Smith

Preop. Dx Cholecystolithiasis OR nurses Jones / Rikes

Postop. Dx Same

Operation Cholecystectomy c̄ C.D. Exploration

Drains T-Tube - 1/2" Penrose Culture 7/30 Results Staph. aureus coag + Resistant-amp-Pen

Path. report 8/2 neg.

Preop. visit 7/26 Postop. visit 7/30

Date	Temperature	Medication	Condition
7/28	100⁶	Demerol 100 x 6	Chart review - Pt. had uncomfortable day.
7/29	99⁸	Demerol 100 x 4	" " cond. satisf.
7/30	101²	Demerol 100 x 4	Visited - complains incisional pain. incision red - serous drainage upper canthus - Wound and skin precautions.
7/31	101	Gentamycin	Complains of pain when he coughs. Instructions reinforced - wd. drainage.
8/1	100	"	No complaints - wd. draining ambulatory in room.
8/3	99	"	Cond. satisf. may go home tomorrow

Name Ray Wilkins Room 640 Date of surgery 7/27

Fig. 9-1. Completed postoperative visit card.

POSTOPERATIVE INFORMATION CARDS

Although any system of record keeping can be utilized, a suggested method is the use of 5 by 7 inch cards, which can be filed in a Kardex system. The nurse can easily refer to these cards and can use them on postoperative visits. Fig. 9-1 illustrates a completed postoperative card.

A clerk or nurse in the operating room can fill in the top portion and the bottom line of the card on the day of surgery. These cards can then be filed according to date; each day the nurse completes the card for that day with information taken from the chart or observations made while talking with the patient. The card is then placed into the next day's slot. This is done on a daily basis until the patient is discharged or has made a satisfactory adjustment to his condition. After the patient is discharged, the cards can be kept for a period of time and utilized in various ways.

SITUATIONS AND COMPLICATIONS ENCOUNTERED
DURING THE POSTOPERATIVE VISIT

As the operating room nurse begins the postoperative visit, she first checks the patient's chart and from this, fills in all pertinent data on the patient card. A conference with the unit nurse will disclose the existence of any behavioral problems. The operating room nurse is then ready to visit the patient.

It is important that the nurse reintroduce herself to the patient. Although the majority of patients will remember her, some, because of sedation or other drugs, will have difficulty placing her among the myriad of people who have been attending to them.

Those patients who do remember will usually respond to the introduction with some comment about how they have been following instructions. (Nurses in the postanesthesia room tell of patients who are heard inhaling and exhaling deeply while recovering from anesthesia. If the recovery room nurse asks them what they are doing, they will usually say, "clearing out my lungs," or "deep breathing exercises." This may occur at a time when the patient is not yet lucid enough to identify his surroundings.)

If the patient has had problems with pain, the nurse considers the type of surgical procedure that was performed. The incisional site is then checked for signs of inflammation or infection. If the incision is healing well but the abdomen appears distended, hard, and shiny, the patient is probably suffering from "gas pains." This could be symptomatic of more serious complications, and the supervising nurse should be notified of the situation so that corrective measures can be taken. An overdistended bladder can also cause much discomfort and should be relieved as soon as possible.

Should there be no obvious reason for excessive pain, the nurse should once again (as in the preoperative visit) draw up a chair and listen to the patient as he talks. A casual, unhurried attitude is most important. The nurse can always begin the conversation by assuring the patient that a certain amount of pain is to be expected. She will explain that, as the incision heals, there will be a strain on the skin sutures. The patient feels this strain or pulling, and when the stitches are removed, this pain usually disappears.

The crying patient

Occasionally the nurse, upon arriving at the bedside, will find the patient crying. This is very often an uncomfortable situation. The nurse may feel compelled to comfort the patient by uttering platitudes such as, "Now, Mrs. Smith, it can't be that bad; everything's going to be all right." How does the nurse know that "everything is going to be all right" when she doesn't even know the problem!

Crying is a form of communication. It conveys discouragement, sadness, pain, frustration, anger, or grief. Sometimes it is a plea for help.

Crying may also be an expression of relief or the patient's way of releasing pent-up emotions. The tearful patient does not always know why he is crying and is often unable to give a reasonable explanation for his tears.[1]

The nurse must be able to tolerate crying in others. She must wait quietly until the patient can control his tears for only then will he be able to convey the cause or causes for the episode. The nurse should simply stand by the bedside and place a hand on the patient's shoulder or give the patient a tissue. This, in itself, is supportive because the patient realizes that the nurse understands his feelings and can accept his tears as a perfectly normal phenomenon.[2,3]

The nurse learns to understand the postsurgical patient as she applies learned theories, concepts, and past experiences to the patient's specific behavioral problems. The hospitalized patient is exposed to many psychologic and physiologic stresses. His response may be defensive, which reveals his anxiety in various ways. The nurse must learn to recognize and deal with these manifestations.

Rarely will the patient voluntarily acknowledge that he has a problem. The nurse must learn to look at the behavioral pattern of the patient, for it is by his behavior that the anxious person attempts to resolve the situation that threatens to overwhelm him. The nurse must actively listen and permit the patient to verbalize his feelings.

Disorientation versus postoperative psychosis

Patients who have undergone complex or critical surgery will exhibit symptoms of vagueness about time, place, and person. This is known as disorientation. The disoriented patient needs to be reassured and reoriented. This can be done as the nurse cares for him. The nurse must support the patient in his quest for reality.[1,3]

Postoperative psychosis must be differentiated from disorientation, since the behavior patterns of patients suffering from these disorders may be similar. Whereas the disoriented patient has lost contact with reality, the psychotic patient has feelings of worthlessness and dejection about himself. The psychotic patient's behavior will usually take one of two forms. It will be manifested in either withdrawal or combativeness. Such behavior is exhibited because the patient is frightened and does not feel that verbal communication is an adequate method of expressing himself.

Nursing intervention must consist of providing understanding support. The nurse must maintain authority and remain in control of the situation. External controls are comforting to the patient until he can assume responsibility once again for his own behavior. Nurses must be aware that bizarre behavior, behavior contrary to acceptable standards, is frightening. They will have a tendency to withdraw from the patient whose actions are frightening. This is a poor response and must not be allowed to happen.

One member of the staff should attempt to find the reason behind the behavior so that it can be brought out into the open and discussed in a nursing conference. A plan of action can then be set up to combat the frightening behavior and ease staff anxieties. If anxiety of the staff is not overcome, then mutual withdrawal takes place and the patient loses the supportive care of the one person who can help him make an adequate adjustment—the nurse.[1,3]

The patient who is able to verbalize his fears and communicate his anxieties might seem to be the easiest for the nurse to talk to. Caution is urged that the nurse avoid platitudes and offer sincere help instead. The patient who is extremely ill and uncomfortable simply will not appreciate the nurse who breezily announces, "Now, Mr. Wilkins, let's sit up, the operation is over and you should be feeling just great."

Some patients will want to tell someone what their problems are. They need realistic reassurances; they need someone who will sit with them for a few moments, hold their hand or stroke an arm and listen. Sometimes an answer is wanted, sometimes just a nod of understanding.

Some patients cannot verbalize their fears and anxieties. These patients tend to feel so threatened by illness that they refuse to recognize their feelings. They hide their fear by engaging in aggressive behavior. This is observed in the patient who is excessively demanding and critical of all attempts to care for him. Such a behavior pattern is established by the patient to make him feel less afraid. His behavior is an expression of his inner turmoil and should not be considered as a response to an environmental situation.

These patients should be kept well informed of every procedure to be performed. They need a good deal of the nurse's attention even though their behavior appears to be likely to drive the nurse away. Again, the nurse must be aware of the underlying fear that produces the bizarre behavior, but she must never let the patient realize that she is aware of his true feelings. Then the situation will become intolerable for him.[1]

The depressed patient

The depressed patient is simply reactiong to his situation in the hospital in the same way that he would react to any stressful situation outside of the hospital. Patients who have had radical surgery for carcinoma are likely to experience a depressive syndrome postoperatively. They must not only cope with the usual preoperative anxieties experienced by most patients, but also with the devastating knowledge that they have cancer.[2]

The patient's postoperative response is influenced by his personality and the degree of anxiety he feels preoperatively. The anxiety level of a patient is largely dependent on previous pain experiences. Although pain as such may not be remembered from past experiences, the memory of previous responses such as fear, discomfort, and the inability to control the situation is present in the patient's mind.

Another factor involved in the cancer victim's outlook is the possibility that by cutting out a portion of the body he will be cured. This becomes the focal point of the patient's attention. Conversely, the patient must also consider the possibility that, despite the loss of a body part, he will not be cured and will still face the prospect of death. All of these factors contribute to the likelihood of a postoperative depressive reaction.[2]

The operating room nurse can learn much about the patient's unconscious thoughts by being alert to his choice of conversational topics, descriptive words, and responses to nursing care. If the nurse allows him to talk about his hostilities and refrains from passing judgment, the patient may well avoid a depressive reaction after surgery. Anger, guilt, and anxiety are all present in the potentially depressed patient. The nurse cannot change this, but she can be available for communication. The nurse can also modify the patient's environment so that he can exercise some control over his daily life.[1]

The dying patient

One of the most difficult situations encountered by the operating room nurse on postoperative visits is the dying or terminally ill patient.

Throughout this text it has been emphasized that nurses listen to patients and talk with them about matters of serious concern to them or their families. Death is, of course, a very serious matter. Although death is as old as human beings, few people know when or how to discuss death with a patient. Because our culture is youth-oriented, we are inclined to deny or hide the phenomenon of death. We are uncomfortable in the presence of death and, as a result, most of us are unable to talk with a terminally ill patient with any degree of comfort.[3]

Nurses must look at their own conceptions concerning death and verbalize their own fears and inhibitions. Only then will they be able to analyze their feelings toward the terminally ill patient in relation to themselves. The nurse must also be able to talk meaningfully to both patient and family as they move through the various crises that are associated with the process of dying.

The operating room nurse must not neglect the dying patient while making postoperative visits. The patient may or may not have been told that he has an incurable disease. Most patients, even if they have not been told, are able to sense the prognosis from the behavior of those around them. Some patients who have been told their true condition find the information so overwhelming that they are unable to accept the diagnosis. They regress by using the defense mechanism of denial.

The operating room nurse is in somewhat of a dilemma during the first visit to a patient with an incurable disease. The nurse's reaction will be no different from that of anyone else in the presence of one who is terminally ill. There is an uncomfortable, intolerable feeling that leads to a tendency toward withdrawal, but this must not happen. The dying patient requires extra time and attention. He wants compassion, not pity. The nurse must not appear rushed or anxious to leave; she must make herself available and must convey a humane attitude.

The patient should be allowed to set the pace of the visit. If he denies his condition, the nurse should not try to break down his defenses. Each patient copes with stressful situations in his own way.

The nurse should always be ready to discuss death if the patient wishes. A patient will seldom discuss death as it involves him but rather will discuss it on a philosophical or religious level. The nurses should not attempt to change his focus. When conversing with him, emphasize the present—for him, there is no future. Communications must be kept open. When expression is no longer possible, the opportunity for supportive nursing care is lost.[1,3]

POSTOPERATIVE INFECTIONS

Nosocomial or hospital-associated infections occur in approximately 5% of the 30 million hospitalized patients in our acute general hospitals each year, according to reports from the Communicable Disease Center in Atlanta, Georgia.

A 5-year study reported by Cruse, involving 26,356 surgical patients indicated an overall infection rate of 4.8%. Breaking this down into types of wounds as defined by a National Research Council Study, Dr. Cruse obtained the following rates:

Clean wounds: Those wounds in which the surgeon did not enter the gastrointestinal or respiratory tract. There was no inflammation and no breaks in aseptic technic. The incidence of infection based upon 20,092 cases was 1.8%.

Clean contaminated wounds: Those incisions through which the gastrointestinal or respiratory tract was entered but with little or no spillage. Based on 4,557 cases, the incidence of infection was 8.9%.

Contaminated wounds: Operations where acute inflammation without pus formation was encountered or there was no gross spillage from a hollow viscus. Nine hundred four cases had an incidence of 20.9% infection.

Dirty wounds: Those operations in which pus or a perforated viscus was present; 803 cases showed a 38.7% incidence of infection.

The Joint Commission on the Accreditation of Hospitals in the United States recommends that hospitals with 250 beds or more utilize the services of an Infection Control Officer. Many hospitals have placed a registered nurse in this role, who serves as a liaison person between the Infection Control Committee and the nursing staff and other departments in the hospital to relay information from this committee.

The operating room nurse can, by closely working with the infection control nurse, provide surveillance of postoperative nosocomial infection rates for operating room quality control reports. The operating room nurse making postoperative visits is in a position to examine the patient and to recognize clinical symptoms of postsurgical complications, including sepsis. The Center for Disease Control has listed the criteria for identification of nosocomial infections, and most hospitals have adopted this criteria or have devised criteria of their own. The operating room nurse can, by notifying the infection control nurse, speed up case identification.

The infection control nurse can retrieve instant information by utilizing the postoperative visit card to get the data relevant to the investigation. Fig. 9-1 indicates that Mr. Wilkins had an elevated temperature of several days' duration, indicating that there might be a causative factor other than the trauma of surgery. Three days after surgery his wound started draining. Was this normal bile drainage through the Penrose drain, or was it draining from another site? The next day indicated that purulent drainage was cultured and, when the culture report indicated *Staphylococcus aureus* organisms, the nurses knew they had a wound infection with which to deal.

Through the use of the postoperative visit card, the patient's chart, and the operating room log, the nurses can extract information that may indicate causal factors, such as the appearance of several wound infections in what is known as a "cluster." That means that all of the infections appear on one ward, in one time sequence, in one operating room, or in procedures involving the same operating team or specific portions of it, such as the same surgeon, nurses, or anesthesiologist. Walter reports on carriers of *Staphylococcus aureus* among operating room personnel as follows: surgeons—33%; nurses—21%; anesthesiologists—57%; orderlies—71%. He reported on 256 infections in 2,000 consecutive anesthetics attributable to one anesthesiologist.

Postoperative wound, urinary tract, and respiratory tract infection are primary hazards to the surgical patient and, when infections occur, every effort must be made to identify probable causes and then enlist the aid of all personnel to eliminate or correct the causative factor.

When the operating room nurse and the infection control nurse work together with a commonality of purpose, the possible ramifications will be limitless in contributing to quality patient care.

One such possibility extends into the operating room suite. Personnel in the area tend toward the perpetuation of ritualistic dogma. This "we've always done it this way" syndrome indicates a lack of basic knowledge concerning the epidemiology of the infectious disease process. The operating room nurse may enlist the aid of the infection control nurse to assist the staff in updating its knowledge to acquire a better understanding of the principles involved in the transmission of infection. These nurses can then get on with the business of establishing a safe environment for the patient.

SUMMARY

It has been demonstrated how the operating room nurse, as a specialist, can participate in all phases of the patient's care. The first step in postoperative involvement is for the nurse to make a reassessment of the traditional, "we've always done it this way," philosophy, regarding work habits. Then the nurse, as a clinical expert, makes a determination to fulfill obligations to the patient. It is important that the nurse view the entire spectrum of care—presurgery, operative, and postsurgery. The operating room nurse has special talents and is able to communicate with the patient as an authority on the one subject that the patient is most anxious to hear about—his surgery. Following surgery the nurse is qualified to assess nursing needs of the patient and assist the unit nurse to set up a plan of care specifically designed to met the patient's particular needs. In order to reach this goal, the operating room nurse must join forces with her nurse colleagues in the institution and establish an ongoing, mutually agreed upon preoperative and postoperative teaching program for the patient. Continuity and quality of care can be assured only by planning and implementation.

REFERENCES

1. Robinson, L.: Psychological aspects of the care of hospitalized patients, Philadelphia, 1968, F. A. Davis Co., Chapters 4-7.
2. Ujhely, G. B.: What is realistic emotional support? Am. J. Nurs. 68:758-762, April 1968.
3. Benoliel, J. Q.: Talking to patients about death, Nurs. Forum 9:254-267, 1970.

SUGGESTED READINGS

Bocock, E. J.: Microbiology for nurses, ed. 4, Baltimore, 1972, Williams & Wilkins Co.
Change in OR practice lowers infection rates, OR Reporter 8(5) : June 1973.
Garner, J. S.: Nurse epidemiologist instrumental in infection control, AORN J. 20:261-275, Aug. 1974.
Hampe, S. O.: Needs of the grieving spouse in a hospital setting, Nurs. Res. 75:113-119, Mar.-April 1975.
Infection control in the hospital, ed. 3, 1974, American Hospital Association, Visual Images, Inc.
Isolation techniques for use in hospitals, ed. 2, United States Department of Health, Education and Welfare, Public Health Service, Washington, D.C., 1976, United States Government Printing Office.
Kubler-Ross, E.: On death and dying, New York, 1970, Macmillan, Inc.
Lambertson, E. C.: Current nursing education and practice, Conference for Representatives of State Medical Societies Liaison Committee with Nursing, Chicago, 1967, American Medical Association.
National Academy of Sciences, National Research Council: Postoperative wound infections; the influence of ultraviolet irradiation of the operating room and of various other factors, Ann. Surg. 160(Suppl.):1-192, 1964.
Norris, C. M.: The work of getting well, Am. J. Nurs. 69:2118-2121, Oct. 1969.
Robson, M. C., Krizek, T. J., and Heggers, J. P.: Biology of a surgical infection, Curr. Probl. Surg., Mar. 1973.
Rothberg, J.: Dependence, anxiety, and surgical recovery, Nurs. Sci. 3:243-256, Aug. 1965.
Turner, C., and Mahoney, R. F.: After hospitalization, Am. J. Nurs. 64:137-139, Sept. 1964.

Walter, C. W.: Carrier on the surgical team plays major role in infections, Hosp. Topics, Oct. 1969, pp. 123-130.

Weiler, M., Sr.: Postoperative patients evaluate preoperative instruction, Am. J. Nurs. 68:1465-1467, July 1968.

Weisenberg, M.: Pain: Clinical and experimental perspectives, St. Louis, 1975, The C. V. Mosby Co.

CHAPTER 10

EDUCATION FOR OPERATING ROOM NURSING

EDUCATIONAL PATTERNS

As has been brought out in this book, many tasks performed in surgical therapy are technical; other functions are behavioral in nature. Both are components of operating room nursing. Performance of these tasks requires many years of preparation on the part of each professional and varying amounts of training on the part of each nonprofessional. The average surgical team (surgeon, anesthesiologist, nurse, and technician) represents a combined post-high school education and training period of over 26 years. Acquiring this necessary education is becoming increasingly important because quality of care has become a high priority throughout the nation. On-the-job, hit-or-miss training programs in the operating room are no longer justifiable. Thorough and well-organized educational programs in the care of surgical patients are the responsibility of every institution that prepares members of the surgical team. In addition, as the surgical technics become more complex, more time is required to become proficient.

The increasing cost and length of time needed to provide quality education for health care are a major concern in the United States. Newer, more economical ways are being sought to solve this problem. Government supported health care systems are evolving, which will begin to add the dimension of *health* care to traditional *medical* care, because the cost-effectiveness of illness-prevention has been shown to be significant in reducing total health expenditures. The training of health-related professionals of many new types assumes greater importance as roles in health maintenance emerge and traditional medical practice is augmented by a variety of ancillary primary care providers.[1]

Although a number of intermediary health care roles originated as creative solutions to unmet needs during the haphazard development of the 1960s, this trend has given way to a more disciplined awareness of the need for sufficient education and training to assume much greater responsibility for patient care.

Let us assume that operating room skills are learned on a continuum from zero knowledge to complete knowledge of every conceivable detail for every procedure. Practically speaking, it would be desirable to establish at least two levels of operating room staff functions: the technician, generally assigned to the scrubbing role, and the professional, generally given leadership responsibility. This, of course, does not include the ancillary staff who are not directly responsible for patient care.

The technician's knowledge of procedures and instruction is reliable, but not necessarily based on an understanding of the physiology and psychosocial functions in health and disease. Usually unlicensed and with limited communication skills, the technician is best utilized in scrubbing duties under direct nursing supervision. The technician is not permitted circulating responsibility, since he or she has neither the license nor the education to be directly accountable for patient care. Utilization of operating room technicians for direct patient care responsibility (that is, circulating) is contrary to recommendations of HEW regulations and the Joint Commission on Accreditation of Hospitals.[2] The hospital may lose accreditation if this substandard practice occurs. The operating room nurse is responsible for the patient throughout surgery and for the activities of the technical staff to organize and provide direction toward the surgical therapeutic goals of patient care.

Programs for training operating room technicians are not generally standardized or accredited as are professional programs. The operating room technicians, nursing assistants, licensed vocational nurses, and other ancillaries are not educationally or professionally prepared for direct patient responsibility. The lack of standardization, certification, licensure, and role definition of technicians in the operating room has been a serious problem. Only in the military services has the hospital corps trainee been given standardized course work in conjunction with clear cut advancement in status, pay, and responsibility as each phase of training was successfully completed. As a military subordinate, the corpsman is supervised in every task, although during combat he may be expected to carry out rescue procedures alone. The present goal of both professional operating room nursing and technician organizations is to clarify role functions and to standardize and elevate the quality of operating room skills instruction and surgical patient care.[3,4] The existing methods to bring this about are education, legal change, and salary or status inducements.

The newer physician's assistant programs in many universities are being discontinued since they are medically oriented and require medical faculty to provide teaching and preceptorships. As it is, these medical faculty members are often unable to meet the educational needs of their own medical students even without the added demands of a physician's assistant program. Also, the attrition and general disenchantment with the legalization problems of function of physician's assistants have generated a trend toward wider expansion of nurse practitioner programs with a firm legal basis in revised Nurse Practice Acts in many states. (Nurses are not permitted to carry out orders of a physician's assistant). Medical support and public acceptance of the nurse practitioner in an increasing variety of specialties will provide numerous patient services unable to be given before, because the physician was too overloaded and the nurse not legally permitted to give them. This situation reflects the natural growth of professional nursing and the development of a more adequate background in health sciences education.

The licensed vocational nurse will likely be phased into the 2-year associate degree program since it is not economical to conduct two such similar programs in parallel fashion. The products of each of these programs have become indistinguishable from one another, serving only to confuse the public regarding the different capabilities of the licensed vocational nurse (12 to 24 month program) and the associate degree nurse (2-year program).

At the present time the associate degree nurse, as a minimum patient care practitioner in the operating room, has an open-ended basis for advancing her professional growth and status. She can work, earn money, reinvest in further education toward a baccalaureate, master's, and even a doctoral degree. Unlike the technical nondegree programs that produce a technician with only one limited set of reimbursable skills, nursing programs are an open-ended pathway toward educational advancement with identified stopping points along the way. Nursing is the only health care profession with such a pathway.

The baccalaureate nurse has acquired basic leadership and supervisory skills. Her assignment and compensation are necessarily at a higher level. She is able to scrub and circulate for all general surgery and may be given charge responsibility and basic teaching of students.

Postgraduate programs (both postbaccalaureate and postmasters) are available for preparation of a variety of surgical nursing specialists. These programs usually expand the nurse's basic competence; examples of these specialties are nurse midwifery, cardiac surgical nursing, and neurosurgical nursing.

The master's degree equips the nurse to practice in three more dimensions—supervision, teaching, and research. She may plan or organize educational programs or become an operating room supervisor or clinical researcher.

In general, master's degree programs provide the student additional training in teaching, administration, and research. The operating room staff that prizes quality patient care needs as many of these highly prepared individuals as possible, especially for leadership roles as clinical nurse specialists, clinical inservice educators, operating room instructors, and supervisory personnel.

Independent surgical nurse practitioners work in clinics or with groups of surgeons in private practice to extend their practice, for example in free-standing surgical clinics where minor surgical procedures are done under local anesthesia.

The doctoral degree enhances the research skills gained at master's degree level to the extent of developing creativity and leadership in research design, application, and utilization in clinical practice. Although a young science, nursing has begun to build a firm foundation in the development of research skills in doctoral programs in nursing. The number of nurses with earned doctorates is still only .001% of the total number of nurses. There are approximately 1,400 in the world at the present time. These few leaders have moved to change the perspective of nursing practice. For example, a National Commission on Joint Practice (AMA, ANA, AHA) has formed to develop collegial aspects in health care roles, and there are efforts, through state legislatures, to redefine nursing practice in the light of present academic preparation and development.

EDUCATIONAL PROGRAMS

After the previous discussion of the educational levels of nursing practice above, it is useful to review the types of educational programs presently available and indicate the trends for future educational change. First of all, the traditional operating room nursing course was one quarter or one semester in length in the undergraduate sequence. These programs generally diminished to 1 month or even as little as 2 weeks of operating room observation because of the rapidly expanding knowledge base to be covered in the basic program. At the present time many generic nursing programs integrate operating room nursing concepts into a basic course in medical-surgical nursing. Fundamental principles of asepsis are taught in addition to skills in the three-phase care of the surgical patient (preoperative, surgical, and postoperative, including application of the nursing process in care of surgical patients). In this way the student learns aseptic principles, which are applicable in any nursing situation in or out of the operating room. When properly structured, the course also provides the student with a foundation for later application to a specialization in operating room nursing.

Postgraduate courses in operating room nursing offer organized learning experiences in nursing care of the surgical patient, procedural skills, and anatomy and physiology. These usually take place over a 6- to 9-month period. Some courses offer college credit or continuing education units (CEU's) ; others are given as part of the hospital's education program. Scrub assignments carry somewhat less responsibility and are usually the first skills a student achieves. Thereafter, assignments include circulating, setting up for complex procedures, and finally, taking charge of the suite over weekends, evenings, or nights as competence and skills expand. From 2 to 4 weeks are usually spent studying each major surgical specialty, and there are selected scrub and circulating assignments in each category. (See Chapter 2 for a listing of categories of surgery found to be helpful in delineating student experiences.)

If a student demonstrates exceptional proficiency in a specific type of surgery, this may become the chosen field for specialization when the program is completed. Or the student may elect to remain a "generalist"—able to perform with competence in all general surgical procedures. In addition many courses are offered in operating room management and supervision.

For many students, the first weeks in the real setting of the operating room are frightening. In truth, the problem of providing a well-planned experience for students, based on principles of learning theory, has often been ignored. Classroom lectures might have dealt with topics related to orthopedic surgery, but when the assignments were made, the student was sent to an operating room to scrub for a hysterectomy because that was the room that needed coverage at the moment. It has also been true that not all staff nurses enjoy the responsibility of teaching students, yet frequently students would be assigned to work with these staff nurses. Not surprisingly, there were negative outcomes for both student and staff member. Little effort was expended in paving the way for the students in an integrated fashion by building their knowledge purposefully or by helping them gain confidence. We now know that the student's ego is strengthened by promoting successful experiences and by careful preparation to accept and deal with the crisis-ridden atmosphere of the operating room.[5]

In academic programs today much of the course work in theory and lectures is presented in multimedia fashion (for example, color videotape casettes) so that the student may pace his or her own learning. Modular mediated lessons in specific skills may be repeated until the viewer is competent to perform the skill in a clinical situation. The role of faculty in such a system becomes that of advisor and clinical supervisor with the responsibility to test the student with reliable and valid test formats. This is important because the student and his or her subsequent employer must be certain that the skills and knowledge obtained are indeed within the capability of the student and used selectively and appropriately.

EDUCATIONAL TRENDS

It is of some interest to view the educational trends in nursing as they relate to operating room nursing. Historically, nursing can be proud of the fact that it has provided meaningful education for health care workers for nearly 100 years, and furthermore, has carried its services to rural and underserved areas. The United States Department of Health, Education and Welfare has provided for continued financial support for nurses in graduate study and in nurse practitioners programs in an effort to build the nation's supply of qualified first-line instructors, practitioners, and clinical nurse specialists. Over a 20 year period since the 1950s, the associate degree and technician programs developed to fill an explicit need for manpower in technical, dependent health service roles.[6] In the late 1970s, emphasis has shifted to graduate programs for the preparation of competent clinical specialists at the master's level. As population increases in the United States level off, the crowding of schools has diminished. In many areas, older school buildings are razed and not replaced. In the next decades there may be an adequate number of health workers to meet the needs of the general population. In some disciplines and in some geographic areas an oversupply may already exist.[7,8]

In relation to organization, accreditation, and control of health care services and education, there are state trends toward formation of joint medical, nursing, and osteopathic state boards that also include lay members to represent consumers and to approve educational programs for nurses in expanded roles, in primary care, in assessment and diagnosis, in treatment within clinical specialty areas, in independent clinical activities, and in rural settings.

State legislatures revised their business and professional codes to allow new, but clearly defined and adequately supervised, experimental programs for training health service personnel to be put into effect on a trial basis.[9] New York and California have been leaders in the revision of state **Nurse Practice Acts** to allow for expanding responsibilities for nurses as well as additional responsibility and decision making in respect to patient care.[10] These changes have been hard-won progressive moves to provide a constructive response to public need. The legislatures have transformed this response to public need into law without relinquishing their responsibility to protect the public during the initial development of new roles in health care delivery. Today's operating room nurse is no longer bound by traditional roles. State laws have changed to allow greater responsibility for individual practice and wider application of nursing in health maintenance.

Continuing education

In fulfilling these new responsibilities for health care there is an increasing need for the nurse to be aware of all new developments in her field of practice. Recognizing the extent and importance of the need for continuing education, some states have enacted mandatory continuing education requirements as a prerequisite for relicensure. Other states have proposed voluntary continuing education programs. In order that nurses may have a standardized approach to continuing education, whether in voluntary or mandatory states, the American Nurses' Association will assume responsibility for accreditation and approval of continuing education programs, working with accredited academic and clinical institutions and specialty nursing organizations and state nurses associations. The AORN (Association of Operating Room Nurses) acts as one of the continuing education accrediting bodies for operating room nursing programs and offerings, in conjunction with the ANA.

As might be expected, continuing education divisions in the health sciences are burgeoning in many directions to accommodate the endless variety and levels of clinical practice review and updating. Most faculty members in health sciences provide some portion of their teaching hours in continuing education courses, which may be given in the evening, on weekends, or in special seminars or short workshops. Space in collegiate settings is thus more efficiently used (for undergraduates during the day, clinical practitioners after hours).

Operating room nursing, too, has become a more complex and specialized form of nursing care. Like other nursing specialties, it has developed a body of knowledge and skills peculiar to itself. Although other nursing specialties have developed separate identities and worked toward defining their special functions, the critical need for ongoing education in technical and psychosocial skills is nowhere as great as it is in the operating room setting. Operating room nursing technics are not normally a part of general or any other nursing specialty and so must be supplied by specialists. To fill this need, the Association of Operating Room Nurses, Inc. (AORN) was organized in 1954 and is now the nationally recognized resource for education toward maintenance of quality care of patients in the operating room. The AORN accomplishes this goal through annual national congresses, regional workshops, seminars, and its monthly publication, the *AORN Journal.*

Competency courses

The newest approach to combining operating room specialization with accepted educational goals has been to offer "competency courses" to graduate nurses, either as continuing education programs for CEU's or for academic credit. The educational outcomes for students in these courses are stated in terms of competencies, implying not only conceptual achievement but clinical capabilities the employer may expect to find in the student who completed the course. In this way nurses can continue classroom study in the college setting and still have extended supervised exposure to the clinical setting. The collaboration of the clinical nurse specialist in the operating room, who may function as a teacher in the clinical setting, with the nurse educator in the college who provides basic knowledge of health care services, offers a balanced and coherent program for the student. In addition to offering clinically useful courses for credit, this provides an escape from dead-end training, that is, training that carries no academic credit toward a degree.

Certification

The American Nurses' Association has begun a nationwide program of certification for practicing nurses, based on clinical achievement and expertise. The certification examination is given the applicant in one of five nursing areas: community health nursing, maternal-child nursing, psychiatric nursing, geriatric nursing, and medical-surgical nursing. Operating room nurses are under the jurisdiction of the medical-surgical division and will be given an opportunity to prove themselves proficient in the total patient care responsibility to obtain certification. The certification process of the American Nurses Association is intended to provide a new method of recognizing excellence in both clinical and scholastic endeavors. It may be compared to the American College of Surgeons, which grants fellowships to selected physicians who have achieved expert qualifications in their specialty.

Inservice education

The term "inservice education" describes the programs developed by service institutions that are designed to (1) provide employees and staff personnel with continuing review of new concepts and skills, and (2) motivate the staff to keep informed of recent advances. In their most limited form, the inservice programs are orientation sessions for new personnel and serve to promote the aims of the institution. Principles of care are usually incorporated and explained as they are practiced in the institution. The programs are intended to facilitate the adjustment of the newcomer to the institution and its characteristic work patterns.

Ideally, the inservice education division of the health care facility has links with the continuing education departments of nearby colleges and universities and can invite faculty lecturers to contribute to the training and development of the institution's staff. In exchange, the practicing health professionals of the hospital or clinic are invited to present programs in the educational institutions. In this way students have an opportunity to learn more about the clinical application of theory and gain a clearer understanding of the problems they will meet as graduates in clinical practice.

Well planned inservice education (as a part of a staff development program) for operating room personnel might include periodic presentations detailing the patient care activities that are offered in the rest of the hospital. Speakers might include the hospital's legal consultant, a radiation therapist, and a member of the Board of Trustees, each of whom would explain his function in such a way as to give the operating room staff a broader view of the patient care process. These speakers might also suggest ways in which the operating room staff can improve the total process.

Inservice programs can be planned to involve other services and disciplines so that the breadth of operating room staff knowledge continues to widen rather than to contract into "operating room only" attitudes. Debates on current issues in nursing, group involvement in professional nursing organization activities, and other efforts to improve the caliber of operating room service will provide the staff with diversified interest. If there is a nearby college of nursing, the faculty may provide the inservice or continuing education programs, as stated previously, and offer units of credit of either the CEU type (10 hours = 1 CEU) or regular academic credit (3 semester hours = 1 unit; the student must be registered at the college and pay tuition). If faculty at the college seem reluctant (or unable) to provide these educational services, the qualified operating room practitioner may seek a joint appointment (part time faculty, part time staff), with proportionate salary from each institution, and serve in the role of educator in the operating room setting.

Specialized practitioners in acute care settings or clinical nurse specialists in surgery are usually not limited to traditional operating room skills but have additional competence in pre- and postoperative care, including areas such as recovery room, intensive care, burn unit, delivery or emergency room. These specialties are seen as related or similar to services in the operating room, although specific procedures differ according to setting and purpose. Acute care or surgical patient management is not limited to the operating room, nor are the clinical skills of the operating room the only ones an operating room clinical nurse specialist needs. The ability and desire to teach are among the most important skills of the clinical specialist. Good teachers are not born; they develop slowly and with much time spent in study of literature related to the subject they teach. For this reason, teaching, management, and research skills are best learned in graduate nursing programs.

Audit and peer review

Why mention audit in a chapter on educational aspects? Audit has recurrent implications for practice. Emphasis on evaluation of practice, nurse accountability, and audit requirements for accreditation has taken operating room nurses in yet another direction.[11] The attempt to relate nursing interventions to patient outcomes has brought about a new kind of thinking. The cost to patients for nursing service has always been a part of the patient's room cost, along with his laundry, meals, and other tangibles.

In order to begin to appreciate the value of nursing interventions, the interventions themselves must be identified and studied to see what effect they have on the patient. If certain nursing interventions are proved to be cost-effective, then these are the ones that should be consciously utilized in the given conditions. Quality care measurement then becomes an assessment of the value of these interventions in helping the patient regain independence.

The audit is a blend of three kinds of input: the plan for medical therapy, the related nursing care, and the patient's adaptive reactions in the health care situation. Audits of patient care in the operating room, usually done by peers, have attempted to isolate and measure the results in patient response that may be demonstrated to be the result of nursing care. For example, one outcome criterion might be to maintain a sterile, thrombosis-free intravenous therapy route without infiltration, skin abrasion, allergic reaction, or other complication throughout surgery and until the patient is transferred to another service area. The outcome of care can be visually evaluated and a clear-cut decision made as to whether there has been adequate nursing attention to the intravenous administration route. A complete audit contains as many of these outcome criteria as may be clearly identified to be the responsibility of the nursing service area in question. Whether or not the outcomes are achieved and to what degree provides the basis for a comprehensive audit of the service. Process audits, those evaluating the operating room nurse actions, are also being used and are of value in identifying strengths and weaknesses of overall patterns of care being provided in the operating room.

WHAT IS A PROBLEM-ORIENTED HEALTH CARE RECORD?

> The chief ingredient of a problem-oriented record is common sense. Therefore, it is within reach of any member of the health care team. Problem-oriented thinking leads to the reorganization of clinical records along lines first suggested by Dr. L. L. Weed. Used well, the system can facilitate smoother continuity of care, more efficient storage and retrieval of information, more effective audit and review.

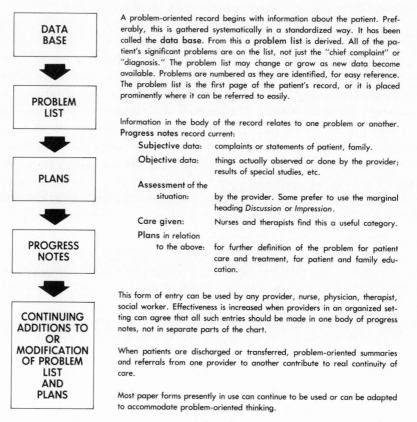

A problem-oriented record begins with information about the patient. Preferably, this is gathered systematically in a standardized way. It has been called the **data base.** From this a problem list is derived. All of the patient's significant problems are on the list, not just the "chief complaint" or "diagnosis." The problem list may change or grow as new data become available. Problems are numbered as they are identified, for easy reference. The problem list is the first page of the patient's record, or it is placed prominently where it can be referred to easily.

Information in the body of the record relates to one problem or another. Progress notes record current:

Subjective data:	complaints or statements of patient, family.
Objective data:	things actually observed or done by the provider; results of special studies, etc.
Assessment of the situation:	by the provider. Some prefer to use the marginal heading *Discussion* or *Impression.*
Care given:	Nurses and therapists find this a useful category.
Plans in relation to the above:	for further definition of the problem for patient care and treatment, for patient and family education.

This form of entry can be used by any provider, nurse, physician, therapist, social worker. Effectiveness is increased when providers in an organized setting can agree that all such entries should be made in one body of progress notes, not in separate parts of the chart.

When patients are discharged or transferred, problem-oriented summaries and referrals from one provider to another contribute to real continuity of care.

Most paper forms presently in use can continue to be used or can be adapted to accommodate problem-oriented thinking.

Fig. 10-1. Components of the problem-oriented record.

Written patient care plans and documented evidence of patient teaching and preparation for discharge are other criteria for evaluating the quality of patient care.

Problem oriented records in the operating room

In order that audits may be made in an organized manner, the chart or record of the patient should be assembled in such a way as to lend itself to this process. The important revision of records into a nationally recognized format[12] brings a greater opportunity to provide meaningful intervention and follow-up to patients whose health histories are organized by the problem oriented method. This method, whether applied to operating room record keeping, or to the entire record of each patient, requires a somewhat different approach to patient care planning.[13] The traditional, chronological, random order of information in patient records is now superceded by the problem oriented format, with problem resolution as the objective throughout the health care delivery process. The Weed system, as problem oriented records were originally called, is well on its way toward universal acceptance, and the implementation of it places increased demands for knowledge and decision making on all health care providers.

The basic components of the problem oriented record are as shown in Fig. 10-1. The operating room nurse's responsibility in contributing to the problem oriented record is to understand the system, its philosophy, and the problem definition, that is, the surgical problem. The operating room must note previously recorded problems that affect the patient's response to the planned surgery and document appropriately the problems that arise as a result of the surgery. She notes problems that may be expected to follow surgery and problems that are *not* expected after surgery, in her follow-up visit to the patient. The problem oriented record thus alerts everyone concerned to the patient's particular set of problems and what is currently being done about them. This type of record provides a rich source for teaching, as well as a ready reference for audit. A typical preoperative progress note in a problem oriented record might appear as follows:

PROBLEM 2:   CHOLELITHIASIS

Subjective: Patient has had severe pain in upper right quadrant for several weeks with nausea, vomiting, burning sensation in throat.

Objective: Gallbladder series taken this a.m. shows multiple stones with lesions at mid-duct.

Assessment: Conservative treatment with diet and Rx has not helped.

Plan: Scheduled for surgery in a.m. Will notify OR and anesthesia resident. Discussed all risks, type of surgery, and expected result with patient and family (wife and son). Operative permit signed. OR nursing staff notified for preoperative teaching and expectation for self-care measures after surgery, i.e., turning, coughing, deep breathing, leg exercises. Please call dietician to see patient 3 days postsurgery to plan dietary intake at home.

Programmed instruction

Programmed instruction is most effective when it deals with limited aspects of technical subjects. It is particularly useful in areas of education in which specific factual content is to be understood by the student. Programmed texts have the advantage of allowing each student to learn at his own pace, correct his own errors, and review whenever necessary without involving other persons in the learning exercise. Topics such as positioning the patient, preparing the operating site, draping, aseptic principles, and anatomy and physiology may best be taught in this manner with the supportive assistance of the instructor to ensure that the content has been learned.

Manual skills are best learned by watching others, either in the actual setting or by videotape or film. Videotaping of various operating room routines or the procedures for setting up complex surgeries, such as craniotomies and open heart procedures, provides consistent, repeatable teaching and refresher information whenever needed. Videotapes can be used by new personnel for orientation or by regular staff members for review. Fig. 10-2 demonstrates how the equipment can be used conveniently by the staff to provide needed information with greater efficiency and clarity.

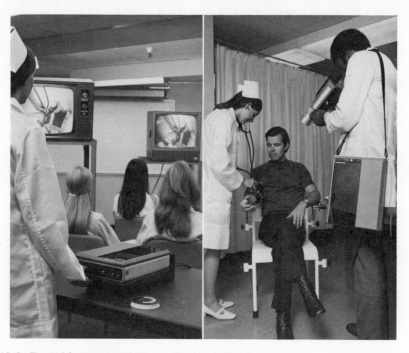

Fig. 10-2. Portable Ampex Instavideo recorder and camera system permits on-the-spot recording of training material. Although blood pressure recording procedures are demonstrated here, this system could be adapted to operating room procedures. (Courtesy Ampex Corporation, Redwood City, California.)

There may never be an adequate substitute for the actual practice of surgical procedures other than the real events. It is nevertheless important to continue motivating more young nurses into the challenge of operating room nursing. These nurses must not be pushed too soon into the arena where they are sometimes allowed to "sink or swim." In the past this approach has caused many young nurses neither to sink nor swim but to "abandon ship" altogether! It cannot be overstressed that the operating room nursing instructor must be allowed to develop the program in such a way as to give each student the time and opportunity to build confidence in his own new knowledge and skills.

There are many ways to use programmed instruction. These programs can be devised according to specific needs of students or operating room staffs. For example, a programmed unit to teach the principles of preparation of the operative site might begin in the following manner.

Frame 1

Human skin is known to harbor many microorganisms which, if they gain access into the surgical wound, could cause infection to occur some time after the surgery, usually within 10 days to 1 month. The purpose of a cleansing preoperative preparation of the surgical site is to remove as many of these microorganisms as possible before the incision is made through the skin. The reason for this is that the scalpel may carry microorganisms from the surface of the skin, where they have remained harmless to the patient, down into the interior tissues where they may be deposited in an ideal environment for growth and subsequent development of infection.

The purpose of cleansing the operative site

with bactericidal solutions is to _____   destroy, remove

as many _____ as possible.   microorganisms

Microorganisms deposited by surgical instruments
from the surface of the patient's skin into the

deeper tissues of the incision may cause _____to appear 10   infection
days to 1 month after the surgery.

Answers to the conceptually graded questions are usually provided at the side of the page or on another page with instructions to cover the answers until an attempt has been made to answer the question correctly with the information provided. Such programs are generally constructed and tested in such a way that they are easily followed in sequence by anyone understanding the language and interested in learning the content. This type of instruction builds confidence in the learner by not permitting failure. If errors are made the first time, they are corrected immediately when the reader checks the answer; in this way few misconceptions can occur.

As an educational aid programmed instruction is inexpensive and useful for teaching many of the operating room routines. This method is time-saving for the instructor and can aid the operating room nurse in understanding many of the physiologic and technical concepts being added to medical knowledge.

ROLE FUNCTIONS IN THE OPERATING ROOM

In the future there may be stabilization among types of health service personnel. Labor unions have been key forces in providing job descriptions for certain categories of ancillary personnel. This, in turn, has clarified some of these roles in the minds of professional personnel and patients alike. However, even labor unions have found it difficult to regulate the hours of work in the operating room or to specify who shall be given "call assignment" and "overtime" duty. Even they recognize that the noon whistle will not automatically stop the surgery in progress.

The increasing overlap of role functions for health care personnel continues to make it difficult to plan sensibly for the educational needs of the various workers. Career ladders and independent roles are being considered as more efficient ways to train more people in the health sciences.

STAFF DEVELOPMENT

There are at the present time many legal, educational, and professional restrictions placed on nursing and ancillary health professions. Dentists, pharmacists, medical and psychologic social workers, physical therapists, inhalation therapists, and many other ancillary workers recognize that their work is adjunctive to that of medicine. There are specified degrees of freedom for each of these categories, and the workers can make independent decisions based on the probability of harm to the patient and the degree to which such decisions are standard practice in the area or region. Some are given license to practice in the area or region. Some are given license to practice independently (for example, the dentist). The nurse may or may not enjoy a similar measure of freedom, depending on a wide range of variables, including expanded roles and national health insurance.

The nurse in the operating room, compared to the psychiatric nurse or the public health nurse, is probably less able to exercise independent judgment. The physician and the anesthesiologist are usually present, which obviates the need for the nurse to make independent decisions related to the surgery itself. Therefore, to outsiders, the operating room nurse may appear to be routinized and controlled in a very narrow set of functions. In reality, however, the nurse has helped to devise these routines that allow the team to work swiftly, efficiently, and at a moment's notice, and does make independent judgments in relation to the aseptic environment and the patient's safety and comfort. This difference might be more apparent if one were to imagine what might result if ten patients were brought onto a ward without prior notice, and what would happen in an operating room if ten emergency patients were brought in at once. The ward personnel are not prepared or practiced in the art of handling life-threatening emergencies, whereas the operating room personnel are always ready with answers and solutions to most of the predictable life-threatening emergencies.

Development of operating room nursing staff must be accomplished by giving each person opportunity and incentive to extend his capabilities individually and, more generally, by exploring new ways to expand the function and responsibility of the staff, as a whole, to provide more coordinated care for the surgical patient.

CHOOSING AN APPROPRIATE MODEL

As stated previously, today's operating room nurses are not content to be relegated to routines. They want a more significant part in preparation of the patient for surgery[14] because their education has given them sound theoretical bases for interviewing patients and utilizing the nursing process and standards of practice.

The nurse may accompany the anesthesiologist on evening rounds to visit the preoperative patients or may vsit the patient independently to assess, teach, and answer any general questions he may have about his surgery. The nurse will also want to see the patient after surgery to see how well he is responding to the care she helped to plan. This visit is also made to see if changes are needed to improve patient's recovery response or if any follow-through is needed on possible iatrogenic problems. New roles for surgical supervision in primary care settings are also emerging.

Patient care requires training, practice, education, review, and evaluation. These activities mean that nurses must pay attention to their own professional development, improving their own skills wherever it is possible. Nurses may become involved in teaching as well as learning. They need to learn to accept criticism constructively, even though it may be given negatively. Although failure may be discouraging for a time, the nurse persists in developing skills and improving technic as is characteristic of a professional in any specialized work.

The operating room nurse is self-disciplined, but not to the point of locking in on one answer to a question and excluding any other. Systematization need not mean dehumanization.

Operating room nursing is discipline with a heart and involvement with a brain. The operating room nurse is never so foolish as to lose sight of her role as a therapeutic agent; yet never so aloof as to be unable to respond appropriately when the patient asks, "Nurse, can you tell me if I have cancer?"

THE VALUE AND UTILITY OF OPERATING
ROOM NURSING RESEARCH

As mentioned previously, it is apparent that nursing has few established methods by which to judge its own competence, except by a somewhat intuitive evaluation of patient well-being. Can these intuitive skills be analyzed and taught to inexperienced nurses who as yet demonstate little intuition? What is the nature of intuition? Is it a type of sensitivity, empathy, or rapport? How does one develop the skill to sense the patient's inner fears and to answer them without having to directly identify them?

Nursing literature contains research results that have a direct application to patients undergoing surgery.[15-17] Some of these clearly indicate that planned nursing intervention can influence the recovery of surgical patients. Abdellah[18] summarized the need to delineate nursing practice on the basis of nursing research and showed why measured comparisons must be made in order to know when nursing is making a difference.

Studies to define concepts; surveys to establish baselines

The reliance on theory and concept formation becomes a matter of urgency in the attempt to establish patient care baselines and nursing care principles. For example, what *is* emotional support? The words are used frequently in relation to preoperative and postoperative nursing care measures, but what actions are implied in the concept?

Investigators have approached the analysis of the concept "emotional support" from different vantage points to offer nurses a clearer understanding of the concept. Rosillo and Fogel[19] describe the interactive process as a combination of identification and magical thinking, with the supported patient "borrowing" the ego strengths of the supporter. Ujhely[20] sees the process as a threefold theme, which the patient projects to the listening nurse: the content theme (the "what" of his story), the mood theme (his manner as he tells his story), and the interaction theme (the way he relates to the nurse and how he would like the nurse to relate to him).

Using this kind of conceptual understanding, the nurse may plan interviews more skillfully and with greater assurance that the patient's emotional distress will be relieved. The nurse can then provide constructive suggestions for nursing care plans.

Operating room nurses need theoretical foundations for their practice; they also need to have at their disposal more facts of current accepted practices in operating rooms throughout the country. The National League for Nursing's annual numerical summary, "Facts About Nursing," fails to distinguish operating room nurses as a separate group. Instead it lists them along with all other hospital nurses. For this reason it has been difficult to ascertain the numbers of nurses actually working in operating rooms, and what trends appear to be influencing the practice of operating room nursing.

Pursuing the future by the predictions of research

A nurse researcher *cannot* be responsible for patient care.[21] This premise is not an easy one to implement when, for example, the nurse researcher notices a patient endangered by nurse neglect. Ethical standards force her to step in to resolve the difficulty if she can; but, thereafter, the observation cannot be a legitimate part of the research data, since she has biased her own observation.

As nurse researchers become a more familiar sight in and out of hospital centers, the results of their research will begin to establish a sound basis for nursing practice. This has not been true in the past. Research skills in nursing have been slow to develop because of the lack of research training among nurses generally. Newer recommendations for nursing education at the graduate level include training in research in order to develop and test the body of knowledge useful to nursing.[22]

EPILOGUE

It is with sincere belief in the following statements that the authors join with nurse educators in the conviction that new ways can be devised to provide all students of nursing the important concepts to be learned from the operating room environment. Even if new technics such as laser surgery and genetic manipulations were to completely replace the familiar technics of the present and the surgical tools now being used were suddenly all obsolete, the *operating room nurse* would still be the *most effective instrument* in dealing with *patient care* and patient needs in the surgical environment. For these reasons, it has been our intent to demonstrate new concepts for nursing intervention that can become a part of the routine of the operating room nursing staff—or a function of what may soon be called the surgical nurse specialist.

The technical skills, which in the past were considered "too technical" to be taught to student nurses, and the environment, which has been considered too threatening to be included in the basic curriculum for nurses, are still a part of operating room nursing. But behind the efficient organization for patient care is a knowledge of psychosocial interactions and how they can be used to achieve a good result for the patient. The patient's welfare depends on the process of operating room nursing as presented in Chapter 2—a process that includes both general nursing considerations of the surgical patient and individual, behavioral considerations.

Special care units have emerged in hospitals (1) because of the desperate need to economize on time for the training of personnel, (2) because special and expensive equipment must be allocated to the areas where it is most frequently used, and (3) because of the patient care gains to be realized when all patients with a similar condition can be together. For example, the intensive care unit for severely burned patients organizes all of the care for these patients in one area, including hydrotherapy and debridement and a special operating room for plastic repair and grafting procedures. Coronary care units, shock units, and cancer therapy units are organized on similar principles.

Specialization is forming along new patient care patterns because so many new technologic advances are now available for restoring optimal health and independence to patients who previously were totally dependent on their families or public agencies. The progress in transplant surgery renews hope for those patients with severely diseased kidneys, livers, or hearts, whose lives can now be lengthened. There is hope that more effective methods will be found to restore the quality of life to those who formerly were able to neither live nor die with dignity.

Does this philosophical digression seem incongruous for the operating room nurse? Hardly. The nurse has helped to design the technics whereby these new procedures were made possible. The nurse has also assisted the patient in the preoperative period by teaching him, listening to his questions, and helping him relieve his mind of whatever concerns might be troubling him. The nurse is sympathetic to his fears and misconceptions and realizes that his fear of death is certainly reasonable. The nurse therefore chooses appropriate responses that will reflect not just her concern, but her value of his life and her belief in his eternal worth.

Whatever the patient's personality characteristics, his response to surgery may well depend on the nurse's actions and choice of words during the terribly sensitive and fearful time before surgery. The patient is vulnerable; his defense mechanisms are being tested, perhaps to their ultimate capacity. He may act childishly; he may cry or be angry, hostile, accusing, evasive, silent, detached, or sleepy. The operating room nurse knows all of the possible defense mechanisms and responds to each with steadying phrases that are carefully designed to help the patient encounter the surgical procedure with the knowledge that this nurse is his ally who will defend him, whether he is conscious or anesthetized, against his own fears and other dangers he may not even understand.

A nurse of this caliber achieves this capability only through experience in operating room nursing. This is not to say that the technicalities of the surgical procedure must be learned before a nurse can be of supportive assistance to the patient; rather the operating room nurse is the only nurse who can comprehend both the physiologic and the psychologic effect of the surgical procedure upon the patient and can plan suitably for nursing care. This care must include all of the expected postoperative considerations and the unpredictable consequences that may ensue. For example, the operating room nurse would understand why a patient's kidney was removed when an abdominal exploratory laparotomy had been scheduled. The surgeon and his assistants will, of course, explain to the patient why the kidney had to be removed. The patient and his family, however, may be devastated by the fact that an unexpected change in the original surgical procedure became necessary once the surgeon could examine the abdomen. If the unexpected actually occurs at a time when the patients' fears are already at a high peak, the psychologic effects may actually delay healing. The operating room nurse knows how difficult this unexpected adjustment may be for the family as well as the patient. Therefore it is this nurse who has the most complete understanding of the probable nursing problems and who can write the best nursing care plan for the patient.

Denial of this fact by educators and the reluctance of operating room nurses who do not wish this added responsibility have diminished. Criticism of the operating room nurse has now become less vocal. There is a great opportunity for the operating room nurse to become a preoperative and postoperative link in the planning of patient care. The operating room nurse may even become involved in discharge planning and instruction for the patient and his family.

Continuity of patient care must become a prime target for interaction planning of every kind of in-hospital nursing service. Continuity is essential in order to make the best use of discharge planning services and public health, family service, and all other services available to patients with health needs.

In summary, this book has attempted to help the reader to become an integral part of the advancing world of operating room nursing. More of everything will be required of operating room nurses of the future: more education, more expertise, more experience, and more preparation for teaching. However, old-fashioned attitudes such as dedication and professionalism have never gone out of style in operating room nursing. Whatever the confusion of the present regarding role functions, the operating room nurses of the future will be the key to integrated surgical therapy for the patient.

REFERENCES

1. Enthoven, A. C.: Can we control the cost of health care? Stanford Magazine 3:14-19, Fall/Winter 1975.
2. Condition of participation, hospitals, Federal Health Insurance for the Aged (Code of Federal Regulations, Title 20, Chapter 3, Part 405), Washington, D.C., United States Department of Health, Education and Welfare, Social Security Administration.
3. Roberts, M., and others: Technicians or nurses in the O.R.? AORN J. 20:466-472, Sept. 1974.
4. AORN and ANA Division on Medical-Surgical Nursing Practice: Standards of nursing practice: Operating room, Kansas City, Mo., 1975, American Nurses' Association.
5. Minckley, B.: Our students wear white hats, AORN J. 8:62-70, Nov. 1968.
6. Montag, M.: Community college education in nursing, New York, 1959, McGraw-Hill, Inc.
7. Edwards, C. C.: A candid look at health manpower problems, J. Med. Educ. 49:19-26, Jan. 1974.
8. United States Department of Health, Education and Welfare, Division of Nursing: The supply of health manpower, Washington, D.C., Dec. 1974.
9. deTornyay, R.: Experiments in the use of health manpower. (Statement of the California Nurses' Association to Assembly Committee of Health and Welfare Concerning the Physician's Assistant.) California Nurses' Association, Dec. 4, 1969, p. 5.
10. Kelly, L. Y.: Nursing practice acts, Am. J. Nurs. 74:1310-1319, July 1974.
11. AORN Committee on Nursing Audit: Nursing audit: Challenge to the operating room nurse, Denver, 1974, Association of Operating Room Nurses.
12. Weed, L. L.: Medical records, medical education, and patient care, Chicago, 1969, Year Book Medical Publishers, Inc.

13. Hurst, J. W., and Walker, H. K.: The problem-oriented system, New York, 1972, Medcom Press.
14. Trail, I. D.: O.R. nurse as a primary care agent, AORN J. 22:118-120, July 1975.
15. Minckley, B.: Physiological and psychosocial responses of elective, surgical patients, Nurs. Res. 23:392-401, Sept.-Oct. 1974.
16. Lindeman, C. A.: Nursing intervention with the presurgical patient, Part 2, Nurs. Res. 21:196-209, May-June 1972.
17. Lindeman, C. A.: Nursing intervention with the presurgical patient. Part 1, Nurs. Res. 20:319-332, July-Aug. 1971.
18. Abdellah, F.: Overview of nursing research: 1955-1968, Part 1, Nurs. Res. 19:6-17, Jan.-Feb. 1970: Part 2, Nurs. Res. 19:151-162, Mar.-April 1970.
19. Rosillo, R. H., and Fogel, M. L.: Emotional support, Psychomatics 11:194-196, May-June 1970.
20. Ujhely, G. B.: What is realistic emotional support? Am. J. Nurs. 68:758-762, April 1968.
21. American Nurses' Association: The Nurse in Research: ANA guidelines on ethical values, Pamphlet D-31, New York, 1968, American Nurses' Association.
22. National Commission for the Study of Nursing and Nursing Education: Summary Report and Recommendations, Am. J. Nurs. 70:279-294, Feb. 1970.

SUGGESTED READINGS

Abdellah, F.: Better patient care through nursing research, New York, 1965, Macmillan, Inc.
Active student participation in the operating suite, Resolution adopted by the House of Delegates, National Student Nurse Association, Twenty-second Annual Convention, April 25-28, 1974, Salt Lake City, Utah.
Aydelotte, M. K.: Issues of professional nursing: The need for clinical excellence, Nurs. Forum 7:72-86, 1968.
Bates, B.: Doctor and nurse: Changing roles and relations, New Engl. J. Med. 283:129-134, July 16, 1970.
Cassem, N. H.: What is behind our masks? AORN J. 20:79-92, July 1974.
Cherescavich, G.: Open forum: Shortage or misuse of professional nursing skills? Nurs. Forum 9:224-233, 1970.
Cooper, S. S.: Continuing education: An imperative for nurses, Nurs. Forum 7:89-97, 1968.
Cooper, S. S., and Hornback, M. S.: Continuing nursing education, New York, 1973, McGraw-Hill, Inc.
Ellison, D.: The need for operating room experience in the education of a professional nurse, AORN J. 3:57-64, March-April 1965.
Gruendemann, B.: Evaluating nursing care: An interim AORN report, AORN J. 20:232-236, Aug. 1974.
Gruendemann, B.: Nursing students in the operating room, Nurs. Outlook 11:129-131, Feb. 1963.
Gruendemann, B. J., and others: Operating room nursing in the basic curriculum: An opinion, Nurs. Outlook 18:44-45, Jan. 1970.
Hunter, A. R.: Nursing audit pinpoints needs, AORN J. 20:241-244, Aug. 1974.
Levine, M. E.: Renewal for nursing, Philadelphia, 1971, F. A. Davis Co.
Litwack, L.: A system for evaluation, Nurs. Outlook 24:45-48, Jan. 1976.
Marram, G. D., Schlegel, M. W., and Beves, E. O.: Primary nursing—a model for individualized care, St. Louis, 1974, The C. V. Mosby Co.
Metzger, N.: Scientific approach to job evaluation, Hosp. Top. 45:37-42, Dec. 1967.
Nolan, M. G.: A master nurse clinician for intraoperative care, Nurs. Clin. North Am. 10(4):645-653, Dec. 1975.
Popiel, E. S.: Continuing education: Provider and consumer, Am. J. Nurs. 71:1586-1587, Aug. 1971.
Popiel, E. S.: Nursing and the process of continuing education, St. Louis, 1973, The C. V. Mosby Co.
Pounds, E., and Askins, B. E.: Criterion-referenced teaching and testing, AORN J. 21:862-866, April 1975.

Ramphal, M.: Peer review, Am. J. Nurs. 74:63-67, Jan. 1974.

Reinkemeyer, A.: End to anti-education bias key to nursing future, AORN J. 19:911-930, April 1974.

Schick, D.: Steps for evaluating patient care, AORN J. 20:237-239, Aug. 1974.

Schlotfeldt, R. M.: Planning for progress, Nurs. Outlook 21:766-769, Dec. 1973.

Smith, K. M.: A rationale for learning experiences in the operating room, AORN J. 4:84-89, Sept.-Oct. 1966.

Stricker, A.: Guard against vulnerability by knowing self and job, AORN J. 20:75-78, July 1974.

INDEX

184